Praise for *The Stark Naked 21-Day Metabolic Reset*

"Brad has completely changed the way I feel, look, and live my life. He gave me the tools to get stronger and healthier and to perform at a higher level. Brad has raised the ceiling of my athletic ability and taught me a lifestyle to make it sustainable."

—BRENDAN STEELE, PROFESSIONAL GOLFER, PGA TOUR

"Not only did I lose 14 pounds in 21 days on the Stark Naked Metabolic Reset but the improvements with my sleep and the energy I gained to thrive every night in my busy kitchen were priceless."

—AMAR SANTANA, CELEBRITY CHEF

"I thought I knew what eating healthy was until I started working with Brad. It's amazing how much better I look, but more importantly how much better I feel, since Brad taught me how to eat and take care of myself. In a profession where my body is my biggest asset and it takes a beating, I feel better in year six than I did in year three. I can't thank him enough."

—ZANE BEADLES, GUARD FOR THE JACKSONVILLE JAGUARS

"Brad's nutrition and conditioning program helped me get back to my season playing weight by reducing my body fat 4 percent in just six weeks. My body feels strong and is free from pain. It's important for a professional athlete to train hard, and Brad is an advocate of hard but also 'smart,' which is why I felt my best heading back to Oakland for my upcoming season."

—LATAVIUS MURRAY, RUNNING BACK FOR THE OAKLAND RAIDERS

"In preparation for Miss USA, I joined Stark Training to get into shape for the biggest competition of my life. Brad and I agreed that the goal was to have a toned yet feminine physique, and that's exactly what we achieved in a matter of a few months. I felt incredibly confident in my bikini on stage in front of millions, and that's a powerful statement!"

—Natalie Pack, Miss California USA 2012

"Brad's Metabolic Reset played a huge role in helping me lose weight and regain energy while recovering from a horrific knee injury."

—Sam Baker, offensive tackle for the Atlanta Falcons

"Brad gives you the knowledge to take care of your most valued asset, your health. Your body is continually breaking itself down and building itself back up. The bottom line is that Brad's Stark Naked 21-Day Metabolic Reset will enhance and perfect this process. This in turn will enable your body to become an efficient fat-burning machine. I don't care if you are twenty-seven or seventy-seven, this plan works!"

—Dr. David C. Roum, owner of D.R. Physical Therapy

THE STARK NAKED
21-DAY METABOLIC RESET

THE STARK NAKED 21-DAY METABOLIC RESET

EFFORTLESS WEIGHT LOSS,
REJUVENATING SLEEP,
LIMITLESS ENERGY, MORE MOJO

BRAD DAVIDSON

WITH LAURA MORTON

HarperOne
An Imprint of HarperCollinsPublishers

HarperOne

FIRST EDITION

Designed by Terry McGrath

Library of Congress Cataloging-in-Publication Data
Davidson, Brad, (Fitness professional)
The stark naked 21-day metabolic reset : effortless weight loss, rejuvenating sleep, limitless energy, more mojo / Brad Davidson with Laura Morton.
    pages cm
Includes index.
ISBN 978–0–06–236921–5 (hardback)
1. Weight loss. 2. Metabolism—Regulation. I. Morton, Laura. II. Title. III. Title: Stark naked twenty one day metabolic reset.
RM222.2.D358 2015
613.2'5—dc23

                          2015024208
15 16 17 18 19   RRD(H)   10 9 8 7 6 5 4 3 2 1

*This book is dedicated to my
beautiful wife, Maria, and my
amazing children, Joseph, Isabel, and
baby Gavin, for their support, sacrifice,
and belief in my crazy pursuits.*

*To my parents, Mike and Rose Davidson,
for grinding every day of my younger years
and giving me the opportunity and security
to take risks and pursue my dreams!*

Contents

Preface

AT THIRTY-TWO YEARS OLD, I looked in the mirror and saw the body I had always wanted and strived for. However, despite looking outwardly amazing, I was keeping a dark secret that was eating away at every fiber of my being. This burden weighed heavily on me day and night.

You see, I was living a totally fake life. On the outside I was the picture of health, and yet I was the furthest thing from being healthy.

Yeah, I looked great, but I felt *horrible*.

Sure, I had those amazing six-pack abs, but I couldn't get going in the morning or function throughout the day without a steady supply of caffeine pumping through my veins. I was severely lethargic and irritable. My thinking was sluggish and foggy. And though I was physically exhausted during the day, I was totally wired at bedtime, so at night I couldn't sleep. Not a wink. To top it off, my sex drive was completely gone.

I could no longer handle my lack of integrity, my daily pursuit of hiding behind my physical image, and my continuously feeling awful on the inside while promoting healthy living as a personal trainer. Overnight, I realized that everything I had learned, believed, and stood behind for so many years as "the truth" in the world of health and fitness had misled me to my harsh reality.

As a fitness professional, I was petrified I would lose my clients, my business, and my reputation as one of the leading trainers in Southern California if anyone found out how weak and tired I felt. I hid my dirty little secret from my colleagues and clients as best I could. I couldn't hide it from my wife, though. When I wasn't working, she bore the brunt of my mood swings.

Of course, my doctor's solution was prescribing the use of hormone replacement therapy and medical drugs like Lipitor to reduce my symptoms and the risk of early death.

Early death! What was wrong?

My doctor diagnosed me with andropause (male menopause). I felt so ashamed and disappointed in myself the day he told me that, at thirty-two, I had the testosterone levels of an eighty-year-old man. For a guy who made a living as a fitness professional, this was a real punch in the gut. From where I stood, it was as if I had hit rock bottom. To be sure, my belief system about health and fitness—that looking fit equaled health—was *completely* shattered.

I meet people daily who are stuck living my old life. They struggle with low energy, are inexplicably overly emotional, are unable to sleep or have interrupted sleep patterns, lack a desire for sex (even if they don't talk about it), and battle to keep their bodies looking great despite hitting the gym 5 days a week.

I imagine many of you might be familiar with this feeling, you know, hiding your true self from the world. Pretending to be bulletproof, invincible. Saying everything is great when it isn't. I hear it from my clients all the time.

Can *you* relate to any of these frustrations?

If you're anything like me, you're probably strong enough to keep yourself from eating too many calories.

You're certainly strong enough to force yourself to exercise harder or more often, even when you don't feel like it.

You're definitely strong enough to avoid carbs at all costs.

And, by God, you're strong enough to suffer through the latest juice-cleanse craze . . . just to prove you can or because all your friends are doing it.

But I have a really important question for you: *Are you strong enough to follow in my footsteps and do what it takes to get your health and your life back?*

To truly get my health and life back it took *vulnerability*. Yup. Vulnerability to admit that maybe I didn't know it all—and maybe, just maybe there is a better way of life. Vulnerability to humbly ask for help, and then to be open to exploring different ideas I thought were foolish at first, but ones I was willing to try if it meant healing myself for the greater good and for the rest of my life.

Yeah, I was more than willing to put myself out there for that.

Over the past eight years, being strong enough to be vulnerable has dramatically improved the quality of my life. But more important to me, it has led to the creation of this program, the Stark Naked 21-Day Metabolic Reset.

Why did I decide to name this program "Stark Naked"?

Simple. In German, the word *stark* means "strong." (That's why I named my company Stark!) And there is no greater form of vulnerability than being naked, is there?

Once I overcame my early andropause and healed my metabolism, the root cause of my symptoms, through the natural methods I share in this book, I made a vow to live my life in the most authentic way. No more lies.

So I am not going to pretend to be an unassailable guru with all the answers. I can only share my journey of what got me healthy and how I've helped thousands of people do the same.

Here's something else you need to know up front.

I am not a medical practitioner or a research genius. I am a top-tier performance coach who works with people on an individual basis and gets excellent results. I won't have the answer for everyone, but it is highly likely that I can help you improve the quality of your life . . . in a very big way.

There is no doubt this book will challenge your current strategies and beliefs, but if you're struggling as I was years ago, that challenge is exactly what you need. It will challenge the rules that have been hammered into your head over the years about what it takes to not only look good, but to feel good too. There are going to be things I ask you to do that go against everything you've ever been told. Be vulnerable and try them. I did, and they changed my life. I just need 21 days to make you a believer.

Before we start you need to ask yourself this important question: *Are you strong enough to be vulnerable enough to step out of your comfort zone and try something new . . . perhaps something that goes against everything you think you know for the next 21 days?*

If the answer to this question is *yes,* you're going to rock this plan.

If you're not sure, put yourself in my hands for the next couple of hours as you delve into my story and the "why" of my program. If I can't convince you of the merit and reasons you should give your body a reset based on what you read, well, maybe you're not ready yet. I hope you'll get there someday. When you're ready, or when you just realize you feel lousy and want to feel better, I'll be here for you.

Here's one more thing to consider. If you are the kind of person who likes to cut to the chase—and you know who you are—you can jump right to Chapter 11 and dive in to the Stark Naked 21-Day Metabolic Reset. Think of Chapter 11 as the "how" and the rest of this book as the "why." The plan has been designed to be easy to follow and ready to do as a self-contained chapter.

Although I'd like to believe that most of you will want to understand why my program works the way it does—especially because it breaks from traditional thinking in so many ways—if you really just want to get started, go for it. No harm, no foul.

If you feel the need to slowly dip your toes in the pool before actually diving in—and believe me, that's going to be most of you—the rest of the book is for you.

Introduction

MY LOVE AFFAIR WITH EXERCISE began when I was in eighth grade. It started the day my father brought home my first set of free weights and taught me the proper way to work out in the confines of my bedroom. Even though the space was extremely limited, I thought, "If *I* can get into shape in this tiny space, *anyone* can!"

My first military presses made me feel as though I was on a teeter-totter, trying to balance my arms and keep the weights steady in my hands. I was terribly wobbly and unsure of myself, but I was immediately hooked on the idea of getting fit! From that moment on, I dedicated my life to looking good and wanting to help others feel better about themselves too. I wanted everyone to feel what I felt.

You see, I was that kid in the eighth grade who started to work on his body right around the time his body was changing, so when I bulked up, got into fantastic physical shape, and was ripped from my arms to my abs, everyone took notice—especially the girls. Man, I liked how that felt!

When I was old enough and able to afford it, I moved to California to pursue the world of physical fitness as a personal trainer. What guy dedicated to his body didn't dream of someday working out on Venice Beach with Arnold Schwarzenegger and Franco

Columbo? I must have watched *Pumping Iron* a hundred times!

Although I loved being a trainer, my true passion for health and wellness was ignited when I was thirty-two years old. As for most of us, it took an awakening—the kind no one really wants to have, but sometimes needs—to understand something's got to give or there will be a significant price to pay in the future.

Okay, I'll come clean. Like so many people in my field, I'd grown a bit overconfident. I was that guy who thought he was invincible—living large, moving at a fast pace, eating what I genuinely believed were all the right foods, and hitting the gym hard. From the outside, I was doing everything right, and yet I felt awful. I had terrible insomnia, and my energy level and sex drive had hit rock bottom. My body was starting to change too. Despite being a top-tier trainer, fat was creeping in around my washboard middle, and I felt weak.

As if that wasn't bad enough, one morning I awoke to discover I was missing patches of hair from my beard. At first, I thought my wife was playing a joke on me by shaving little strips off in my sleep, but she swore she hadn't.

Suddenly worried, I went to see my doctor to check things out. After a battery of tests, he informed me that I was suffering from low testosterone caused by . . . wait for it . . . *stress!*

Stress?

In my early thirties, I was told by my doctor that I was in early andropause (male menopause), brought on from high levels of stress. *WTF!*

My total testosterone level was akin to that of a typical eighty-year-old man. *Huh?*

I knew I was tired, *way too tired* for a guy my age. I could tell my metabolism had slowed down a bit, because I was lethargic and had begun carrying around my waist a new and unwanted thick layer of belly fat—something I couldn't seem to get rid of, no matter how hard I tried (not what you'd expect to hear from a trainer). But I couldn't believe my health had deteriorated that much over the last few years.

I was secretly hoping my clients wouldn't notice my ever-expanding waistline. To hide it, I wore baggy clothes over my love handles, thinking I was being superclever. After all, who wants to work out or take fitness advice from a fat trainer?

There I was, selling health and vitality, and my life was so far from that ideal image. I was such a fraud. When I finally stopped lying about what was going on, I had no choice but to accept my situation for what it was and not what I wanted it to be. My condition couldn't be fixed over a weekend or by just catching up on some much-needed sleep.

Don't get me wrong. That would have been great, but it wouldn't have solved my real issues or been effective for me long-term, because my body was crying out for help. The biggest problem I was having wasn't my testosterone levels. It was that I wasn't tuned in or listening to my body and hadn't been for a long time.

My body was like a computer that had frozen. No matter what I did, all I got was the sad Mac face. What do you do when your computer or phone won't respond?

You reset it!

The harsh reality was that I needed an overhaul—a reset. And since I was aware enough to understand that metabolism is the key to health, I knew I needed an entire *metabolic reset*. (Cue the dramatic music here!)

"Hi. My name is Brad. I was a personal trainer living a complete lie!"

Whew! I feel so much better having this out in the open! Now that I have confessed this about myself, want to know a dirty little secret? Many personal trainers live with this same story. They overwork, overexercise, and don't get enough sleep, because they're trying to keep up with the needs of their busy high-achieving clients. They become experts at maintaining an external image of being fit, when in fact they are just like I was back then—anything but!

The reality is, this affliction isn't exclusive to personal trainers—

lots of people live this way (maybe even you) and don't even know it. And if they do, they're more than likely afraid to do anything about it, because it will upset their "perfect" and "comfortable" routine.

Sound like anyone you know?

When my doctor told me I was sick, I knew the time had come to make some serious changes, but I also knew my usual approach wasn't going to work. My high-achieving, stress-filled, aggressive lifestyle was actually the root cause of my low testosterone and my extreme lethargy, among other side effects, including my low mojo, or sex drive, and weight gain.

But how?

Clearly, exercising hard and eating what I thought was healthy were totally backfiring. *I could not "out-exercise" this new low or "eat" my way to health.*

I had to discover a smarter way to approach my health and reset my metabolism, one that worked for me at a time when I didn't feel like doing *anything*! I needed a solution that could stand up to the stressful demands of my hectic life and work schedule while healing me. Once that happened, my new lifestyle had to prevent another breakdown in my health.

It wasn't easy. There were a lot of starts and stops and lots of trial and error along the way.

I was a human guinea pig, experimenting on myself for months at a time. I experimented with nutritional strategies like eating an extreme Paleo diet, intermittent fasting, and multiple variations of cleanses. I manipulated my exercise protocols, trying high-intensity short-duration exercise, long-drawn-out cardio, corrective exercise, and modified-strongman training. I did extensive lab work testing supplement strategies. I studied functional medicine, obtained advanced certifications in Functional Diagnostic Nutrition, and hired numerous experts in these fields looking for clues to the answers my body needed.

Finally, I found the approach to nutrition, exercise, recovery, and sleep that healed my metabolism, and my andropause reversed itself. My energy was through the roof, my mood was optimistic, my sex drive was back, and, best of all, my body began to look like the body of a qualified trainer again.

And then I had an epiphany. If this plan worked for me, I was certain I could help others with it.

Why?

I had finally found the answers that helped set me on the right path to where I not only looked good, but felt great too. This was what every client of mine truly wanted, but never articulated. As a result of these strategies learned and perfected, I now use this exact system on all of our private clients at Stark, which allows them to experience the same reset and benefits I experienced.

And now, with *The Stark Naked 21-Day Metabolic Reset* these exact same benefits are *yours* for the taking too.

A Lifestyle Plan Designed for You

Finally, there is a lifestyle plan that meets your needs and will help you to live your healthiest life ever, from the inside out. Stark Naked is the only lifestyle plan designed for all of you who believe life is meant to be lived, not just endured, who want to live life on *your* terms!

If you describe yourself as busy, stressed, overcommitted, and tired, you are a person I call a *high achiever.* Don't get freaked out by that term. You don't have to be a titan of business or a guru of greatness to be considered a high achiever.

If you constantly push yourself beyond the limits, have a strong desire to be the best at whatever it is you do, have a drive to be successful, but have become ambivalent about the impact of stress on health, dismissing it as the "price you pay," *you* are a high achiever. If, no matter how much you accomplish, you can't shake the ever present feeling that there are still items on your infinite "to do" list, *you* too are a high achiever.

High achievers can go from being in fifth gear to crashing, and they need 2 or 3 days before they can flip their "on" switch to "off" during a vacation—though they can never really unplug. In general, high achievers are incredibly driven individuals who are in a constant state of stress, focused on a desired outcome, and willing to do whatever it takes to accomplish that outcome. High achievers have an ability to dig in and keep going, pushing through barriers even when everything seems to be against them. Failure is not an option!

Does any of this strike a chord?

It should, because this massive population keeps multiplying and includes young professionals, Gen Xs, Gen Ys, baby boomers, stay-at-home moms, working moms, busy executives, business leaders, law-enforcement professionals, professional athletes, and any others who claim they are constantly on the go.

Could this be *you*?

Three years ago at the age of sixty-three, iconic head football coach Bruce Rollinson, from Mater Dei High School in Orange County, California, stepped into my office to talk about a strategy to revamp his health, energy, and fitness. Why?

He wanted to earn the respect of his players as he demanded that they get more serious about their health. The prior year, his team had their first losing season since he took over as head coach in 1989. It was time for the mighty Monarchs to make a comeback. The coach was tired of seeing pizza boxes in the locker rooms and observing his players not being in top physical condition. He hired a new strength coach to help get the kids into shape. I have so much respect for a coach who leads by example.

When he started working with me, Coach Rollinson weighed 227 pounds. His cardiovascular risk markers were elevated, he wasn't sleeping well, and he really struggled with afternoon energy crashes that were negatively affecting his mood and focus during practices.

To make matters more challenging, he had suffered numerous injuries to one knee that initially limited what we could do in the area of exercise.

In my eyes, Coach Rollinson is the ultimate example of a high achiever—even in his sixties. He's a fierce competitor who was nowhere near ready to walk away and retire from coaching. He still had a lot more games left to win, and he knew it. He just needed some support to reset his metabolism, so his body and energy could keep up with his drive and hunger to keep coaching football.

Within six months, we transformed his body, which dropped 40 pounds. Not only did he reset his metabolism and have the energy to be a better leader; his team totally transformed too! His team ended the next season with an 11–3 record, making it all the way to the CIF Championship game. I will never forget their game at Anaheim Stadium that year against their rival school, Servite High. Coach Rollinson let me bring my ten-year-old son into the locker room before the game, and he got to run out onto the field with the team. Three years later, Coach Rollinson is still going strong. He has kept his metabolism optimized, has maintained his weight, and is keeping his health and energy in check. It's going to take more than age and stress to get Coach Rollinson to retire.

No matter where you are in life, it's not too late to take control of your health and well-being. All it takes is 21 days and a commitment to stay the course.

It's Time to Make a Lasting Change

Get ready for a dynamic shift in the way you think and live.

The Stark Naked 21-Day Metabolic Reset is designed to teach you why you feel the way you do, show you how to reset your metabolism (fix what's broken), and then help you to apply these healthy-living principles to your individual lifestyle. In just 21 days, you will feel great, look fantastically healthy, and perform at an amazingly peak level with more energy than you've ever had or thought possible. When you get right down to it, energy is our greatest asset in this game of life; if your energy isn't up to par, everything suffers.

Today, my schedule is the busiest it's ever been. Not only do I train clients and advise them on nutrition, while traveling the world teaching groups of other high achievers how to reset their metabolism and develop resiliency in their stressful and demanding lives; I also balance those tasks with my responsibilities as a husband and dad. As a result of my time spent perfecting this plan, I can show you how to have that same kind of balance in your life too.

The majority of mainstream diet and fitness advice promises a quick fix, but I have discovered that quick fixes require you to either deprive or abuse the body, in short, to stress out the body. Your body does *not* need more stress. Even when I was diagnosed with andropause and feeling my lowest, I didn't want to believe I was sick. I knew I felt bad, but I still wanted to believe I could work this problem out with discipline and effort. In reality, like you, I was simply exhausted, not sick. My body needed the exact thing I generally considered to be a sign of laziness and weakness. What it needed was the four-letter word *r-e-s-t*!

Say what?

Yes, *rest*.

I grew up with a father who instilled a fierce work ethic in me. He told me that hard work was the essential foundation of success. Quitting was never an option in our house. Neither was being lazy. One of my dad's yearly goals at his job was to win the perfect attendance award. He took so much pride in winning it several years in a row.

In a recent private consultation with a very successful man, our conversation happened to turn to the virtues of rest. He looked at me and said, "Brad, I will be honest with you. I have not taken a full week off of work since I started my business in 1983." Although I am sure this is his secret to becoming hugely successful, imagine the sacrifices he has made physically, emotionally, and otherwise to make that statement.

Now, I realize most of us don't understand the word because we are people on the go, but rest is the magic pill when it comes to health and fitness. High-performance athletes tout the virtues of their off days and the impact that has on their performance. And that's why I made rest and sleep a huge part of this plan. In fact, it's so important to the success of your reset, I dedicate a whole chapter to the benefits of sleep. *Do not skip it!*

Cutting back on exercise when you're physically shot is also important to your recovery, and that's another key element in your reset plan. Believe me, too much exercise combined with one crazy fad diet after another can be a very dangerous thing. In my case, I was actually breaking down my body by trying to combine traditional theories of nutrition (like eating a no-complex-carbohydrate, primarily high-protein clean diet), overexercising, and believing (based on my highly motivated work ethic) that I had to outwork everyone else if I was going to succeed. I wanted to accomplish great things and look incredible at the same time. I got away with that mentality for a while, but slowly that way of thinking and living caught up with me and then *wham*!

I know a lot of you reading this book live life *very* committed to the fire in your belly and accomplishing as much as possible in your life. You likely grew up hearing such sayings as, "You can sleep when you're dead" or "The harder you work, the luckier you get," and perhaps took them literally. That's why you likely work as hard as you do, as a result find yourself in a state of complete fatigue, and think it's actually *normal* to feel that way.

I've got news for you. It's *not* normal to feel this way.

In fact, if you can give me 21 days, I can open your mind, body, and spirit to a totally new "normal." But you've got to be willing to give up your old ways of thinking and try some new things that may rock your world at first.

Hey, I get it. Getting stuck in a rut happens to the best of us. Believe me, I hear it every day. Clients come into the gym and say things like:

"My energy is horrible without caffeine."

"I can't sleep."

"I need to take a sleeping pill to get any sleep."

"I have zero sex drive."

"I force myself to exercise every day, but my body does not reflect my efforts."

"I am looking for answers, and all I can find are the common extreme ones that say I need to sacrifice more and try harder. I need to cut more calories, eat less carbs. I'm not exercising enough or hard enough. I'm supposed to suck it up and try harder!"

"I am at my breaking point!"

"No pain, no gain, right?"

Wrong!

This book will turn everything you think you know about nutrition and fitness on its head and show you what "great" and ultimately "normal" should really feel like. The Stark Naked 21-Day Metabolic Reset is not about healing you from a disease or turning you into a fitness model. If that's what you're looking for, move on to the next fad diet book. I'm not your guy. I'm good at what I do, but I am neither a medical doctor nor a magician.

Besides, looking good but feeling horrible doesn't cut it in my world. Those aren't the results we are after here. This book is a long-term lifestyle plan for those in need of a metabolic reset to elevate their readiness and resiliency, so they can conquer the game of life.

Think of it as a comeback.

Take Control of Your Health and Fitness for the Very Last Time

If you're tired of being tired, sick of being sick, over being under-sexed, starving for better health, and dying to finally live your best life ever—then you are finally ready to take control of your health and fitness for the very last time. Why?

The Stark Naked 21-Day Metabolic Reset is the ultimate tool to build resiliency into your high-achieving lifestyle and allow you to wake up every morning with the "juice"—that necessary motivation—to conquer life one day at a time. Allowing yourself this chance to reset will refuel that inner hunger and drive for being great and getting the most from every day of your life. It will make life fun again!

The reset plan in this book is the exact strategy I use with the professional athletes I train who want to resurrect or extend their careers, the powerful overachieving CEOs who are running on low energy and experiencing unwanted brain fog, and the overextended parents trying to be all things for their kids and suffering from constant fatigue and moodiness.

This book holds the keys to the kingdom. They're yours for the taking. All you have to do is grab them and unlock the door.

You are about to make a paradigm shift. Don't let fear stop you! I have found that most people will go to greater lengths to avoid what they fear than to obtain what they desire.

Here's the thing. Fear kills everything—especially your greatest potential. So often, people come to me afraid of what the future holds—and some, for very good reasons. They've been warned by their doctor that if they don't get a handle on their health, the worst doom-and-gloom outcome is imminent. Frozen by fear, they throw their hands in the air and give up without ever trying. They worry that if they don't get back into shape, their spouse will leave them, they'll get sick(er), they'll miss more days at work, and so on. If . . . if . . . if . . .

Playing a game of "What If" Roulette is a horrible way to live!

I'm here to tell you that *fear is a reminder of what is possible.* Use it to motivate you! This is *your* life. It's not your parents', your kids', or your spouse's. It isn't measured by your job title, your bank account, the car you drive, the watch on your wrist, or even the size of your waistline. It's about being in the moment—the here and now. The master of mindfulness Jon Kabat-Zinn says, "You can't change the tide, but you can learn to surf." That philosophy speaks to me, a California boy, on every level, and that's exactly what I chose to do when I took control of my health and wellness.

Welcome to your new journey, your great comeback! It's not too late to have the life and health you've always wanted.

What You're About to Read

It's important to understand right out of the gate that the Stark Naked 21-Day Metabolic Reset isn't a diet. It isn't a fad. It isn't a quick fix, and it isn't some gimmick that will backfire the minute you screw it up.

Face it: you can't will yourself to feel better. There is no magic bullet. The only true answer is to change your lifestyle by getting healthy and living your best life. In order to do that, you must first fix what's broken. This is the playbook that will show you how to do that.

The first three sections of this book show *why* my program works, including the research and data to support my plan. Part One is all about what has happened to you—what got you to this broken state and why you feel the way you do. It explains the metabolic breakdown process, what caused it, and the symptoms you're likely feeling from it, such as low energy, lack of sleep, zero sex drive, and your body's lack of response to your dieting and exercise attempts.

Part Two explains the massive impact of stress on your body and what you can do to alleviate it. Whether you realize it or not, stress is at the root of your metabolic breakdown. This section of the book is designed to explain the three major culprits that elicit the stress response, causing the Metabolic Breakdown Cycle, *high-achieving lifestyle, toxicity, and food-driven inflammation;* these eventually lead to altered hormones and the ultimate consequence, *total metabolic lethargy*. If these three areas are left out of control, they will eventually destroy your metabolism by first altering your hormones and eventually completely wiping out your metabolism, destroying your energy, body, and desire for life. You can't beat a stress issue by adding more stress. You have to reduce or eliminate it from your routine, and this section will illustrate the reasons why.

Part Three will teach you about the Stark Naked lifestyle and how to get the most out of your 21-day reset. In this section, I will explain why you are going to focus on getting more sleep and why cutting back on your exercise program will help you recharge your broken metabolism and lay the groundwork for your new life as an optimized high performer. I will also give you cutting-edge mindset solutions to help you thrive throughout the Reset. I'm not going to sugarcoat things. The first week can be tough, but this section will show you how to win before you start by helping you buffer daily stress and learning to lead a resilient, optimized life after completing the Reset. Remember it's your current lifestyle choices that have beaten you down. You cannot expect to reset your metabolism and then successfully go back to your old way of living. You have got to fix what's broken and then live a new healthier way of life that supports your reset metabolism—not destroys it.

Parts Four and Five detail how my program works. Part Four is the Stark Naked 21-Day Metabolic Reset. Everything you need for success is in Part Four. If you are eager to start right away, go ahead and jump ahead to Part Four and start rocking. But trust me, as your body and energy begin to transform, eventually you are going to want to know the reasons why my program works, because it defies everything you thought you knew. When that happens, simply go back and read Parts One through Three to learn the "why." You'll be glad you did!

Part Five shows you how to live the Stark Naked life *optimized* after you complete the Reset. Once you feel great again, you won't ever want to return to your previous way of living. The way to an optimized life, in which you have built resiliency into your high-achieving lifestyle, can be found here.

I want you to know that I will be with you every step of the way. You are not alone on this journey, and you don't have to be afraid of the road that lies ahead. I assure you, I've been where you are right now. I know exactly how you're feeling. Together, we will walk this path to better health and wellness and discover what it truly means to not only look, but also feel great.

Are you ready to get started?

Me too!

Let's go!

▶ PART ONE

YOU'RE HAVING A BREAKDOWN

1

You're Having a Breakdown—
a Metabolic Breakdown

"CARBOHYDRATES ARE THE DEVIL!"
      "Eating fat makes you fat!"
      "Do a cleanse!"
"Learn to control your caloric intake."
"Eat more protein!"
"No, wait. Protein kills!"
"Eat vegetarian."
"Go raw."
"Go vegan."
"Go gluten-free."
"Don't eat sugar."
"Don't eat wheat."
"Don't eat dairy."
"Don't eat at all. Just juice!"

Is anyone else confused by all the nutrition and diet information being thrown at us today?

What makes navigating this maze of information even harder is that these "theories," "diets," "plans," and "programs" are each highly researched and, for the most part, backed up by bona fide scientific research by doctors who all tout the health benefits their program allegedly provides.

Worse yet, each program promises to become the next miraculous solution to improve *anyone* and *everyone*.

So who is right? Welcome to my worst nightmare!

If you are bewildered when it comes to eating right and choosing the best foods for you, you are not alone. A 2012 food and health study presented by the International Food Information Council Foundation showed that 52 percent of Americans surveyed thought it was easier to figure out their taxes than healthy eating.

There are so many nutrition plans, diets, and options available, it's no wonder people don't know which way to turn. The biggest problem is that most of the information out there is conflicting! Worse, it's often driven by a larger-than-life personality who has a need to be right. Even if the information being offered has merit, it isn't always geared toward your individual needs. That makes it truly hard to know who to trust or which program is best for you.

And that's a big problem, because what you eat has a huge impact on your health. Everything you're doing to eat "right" is probably wrong.

Fad Diets Aren't the Answer

These days I don't really think of myself as a personal trainer as much as a health and performance coach to many of today's highest achievers and some of the fittest people on earth. In fact, one of my clients, who is the most sought-after real estate coach in the country, refers to me as *his* performance and energy coach! I take that role and title very seriously, because he is a guy who is on the road 230 days a year, speaking to capacity crowds day in and day out, someone who absolutely needs his energy and performance to be at peak levels all the time.

Over the years, almost all of my clients have come to count on me to know about the latest information in all areas of health, nutrition, and fitness, which means I need to be on top of the latest and not so greatest next fad diet that overpromises and underdelivers. They ask me, because most of them want to try it, have tried it, or know someone who has tried it, and so on.

I have sifted through just about every theory, program, and promise *and* the science that backs those diet plans. After going through each from every point of view, I have discovered one very important thing. *Most are not sustainable for long-term success, especially for people like you—the high achievers of the world.*

Although they may initially create some positive results, eventually each one of those trendy fad diets will stop working. Some are actually so dangerous that over time you may actually start damaging your overall health. That's because most nutritional strategies today are designed for the overwhelming number of people who are looking for shortcuts to weight loss, expecting a magic pill to cure their bad habits.

I recently had a client tell me he was considering going on a 15-day juice and coconut-water cleanse.

"Are you moving to Gilligan's Island?" I asked.

He looked at me as though *I* was the crazy person in the room. He was stunned by my straight-faced reaction. I really think he believed juice and coconut water were healthy choices for 15 days. Sure, he might have lost some weight, but the second he went off that diet, he would have put it right back on and wouldn't have earned any benefit for his effort.

"The only reason I can think of to sustain yourself on fruit juice and coconut water for two weeks is if you're stranded on a deserted island," I said.

Seriously, if you are going to put yourself through a program of any sort, doesn't it make more sense to learn how to sustain yourself on a food-based program that you can live by and maintain for the long term? More so, one that has multiple health benefits beyond weight loss?

It's like asking a dermatologist for a remedy for your wrinkles, when your real issue is dry, flaky skin, red blotches, and brown spots. People just can't see past the wrinkles!

People have been led to believe that weight loss is the sole solution to all our health and fitness needs and that because a program makes you lose weight quickly, it's a good program. People who choose a juice cleanse are typically unmotivated to do the necessary work to sustain long-term results. They're looking for a shortcut to weight loss, a magic cure, a quick fix. They're into fad diets, not *health* and *wellness*. They may see weight-loss benefits from the next hot diet plan, but they aren't necessarily getting healthy or creating a lifestyle that will sustain habits to maintain their weight loss. They are merely creating a temporary mindset that achieves their immediate desired result, but no long-term payoff.

For example, if you go on a low-fat diet, you may lose a little weight in the beginning, but in the long run you end up having issues with low energy, lack of sex drive, a sluggish brain, depression, and increased body fat due to a lethargic metabolism. Your brain and your hormones need fat to function optimally. You get the quick initial weight-loss result, but you are trading optimal health for a number on the scale. It's not ideal.

Likewise, removing carbohydrates from your diet creates some weight loss and improved energy on the front end, but if deprived of carbs long enough, the thyroid is guaranteed to struggle and slow down, which will lead to low energy and eventually unwanted fat gain. *Translation: If you're not eating carbs, but gaining weight—now you know why!*

Fad diets are not the answer for people looking for a lifestyle that will sustain both feeling great and looking great. They are not long-term solutions, but simply stressful ways to manipulate your body to quickly force weight off. Here's the bottom line: to obtain long-term weight loss, *you must fix the problem that is causing fat storage* and not damage the body more just to drop numbers on your scale.

Eating "healthy" and working out longer and harder aren't the answers either. I meet so many people who think they're doing everything right and making good food and exercise choices, but realizing zero results! It's so darn frustrating! As a matter of fact, most people start noticing they're feeling even worse as time goes on.

"If I Am Doing Everything Right, Why Do I Still Feel So Bad?"

My client Misty is a thirty-eight-year-old mother of four living in Oregon who was highly committed to eating healthy and routinely exercising, but she was at her wits end because she wasn't getting the kind of results she wanted. Misty is a stay-at-home mom who also works as an onsite apartment manager in the complex where her family lives, so she juggles a lot of responsibility. She paid attention to her diet and believed she was making good, healthy choices about what she was putting in her body. Misty was extremely disciplined, avoided fast food and processed foods, watched her caloric intake, and focused on eating a clean, whole-foods diet most of the time. I totally believe she only put the foods she told me about in her system. Her efforts had rewarded her with excess weight gain instead of a slimmer body. Emotionally she felt so bad, she started taking antidepressants, which only brought on severe fatigue.

During Misty's quest for answers she constantly concluded that she must be eating too much or not exercising enough, because no one could give her another rational explanation for her weight gain. She tried every diet she could find—low-fat, low-carb, and low-calorie—you name it, she tried it. She was willing to try anything just to lose a little weight and feel better.

Her frustrations with exercise were no different. Her only answer was to spend more time in the gym or suck it up and exercise with more intensity. This wasn't an easy task for someone who had to summon up all her natural energy just to get from her bed to the coffee pot in the morning and pray for a kick-start. Caffeine became her lifeline to survive the day ahead of her.

During our first meeting, Misty was shocked when I told her there was no exercise program that would give her the results she was looking for and she should dramatically reduce her exercise commitment every week to start with. I am always amazed at the reaction I get when I first tell new clients that.

"Are you crazy? I will blow up like a balloon if I exercise less."

That's the usual response I hear from people when I tell them this. Misty had fallen hard for the old-school approach of doing more and trying harder to the point of exhaustion. Her body was overstressed.

I did some testing on Misty to see what was really breaking down in her body. Her diagnostic results showed that her liver was overwhelmed from all the coffee she consumed throughout the day and from excessive amounts of exercise. The second thing her results showed was that Misty was experiencing extreme food-driven inflammation. The foods she was choosing to eat were certainly considered healthy foods, but for Misty they were contributing to her problems.

These two conditions were placing extreme stress on Misty's metabolism and causing what I call the Metabolic Breakdown Cycle. Her metabolism had gone into self-protection mode. What Misty needed was to stop the deprivation and exercise abuse and reset her broken metabolism.

It's as simple as this. If I want my car to go faster but I have four flat tires, what will help more? Fixing the tires or pushing the gas pedal as hard as possible to the floor?

You first have to fix what's broken!

Understanding Your Metabolism

After many years of rejuvenating worn-down high achievers, I have discovered the Metabolic Breakdown Cycle. This is the breakdown process that slowly destroys your metabolism and prevents you from experiencing great energy, amazing clarity, a rockin' body, and a youthful sex drive.

Metabolism is one of the most misunderstood of the body's systems. A lot of people talk about "metabolism" and yet few really understand what it is or how it affects health and vitality. This is especially clear whenever I ask my clients what they think metabolism is. Most people say metabolism is the amount of energy a person's body burns or that it has something to do with the thyroid. When I push a little farther for clarity, some say that when the thyroid gets sluggish, they have a slow or sluggish metabolism and that's why they get fat. Although that is all true, over the years I have come to understand that our metabolism is really so much more than that.

Even medical professionals have varying definitions. The classic thought on metabolism is that it is the sum total of all chemical reactions in the body.

However, my favorite definition of metabolism comes from *The Schwarzbein Principle,* by Dr. Diana Schwarzbein and Nancy Deville: "Metabolism is the combined effects of all the varied biochemical processes that continually occur in your body on a cellular level. These processes enable every individual component of your body to function, making it possible for you to think, digest food, move, and perform all the functions of a living, breathing being."

These metabolic processes include such things as hormone production, tissue regeneration, digestion, elimination, and immune responses. In fact, *everything* going on in your body impacts the sum total of your metabolism. If any one of these processes gets a little out of balance, your metabolism pays the price.

Okay, what does that really mean? And more so, what does that mean to you?

For example, if your liver is congested and working on overdrive, it will have a huge negative impact on your metabolism by slowing down your thyroid hormones. Your liver is largely responsible for converting the mostly inactive form of the thyroid hormone, T4, into the active form, T3. It really doesn't matter how little you eat or how hard you exercise; those things won't help your congested liver, heal your damaged metabolism, or prevent the result: unwanted fat storage.

Recent studies have shown that metabolism isn't just a set of automatic physical processes—it's also affected by the emotional connection between the mind and body. What we think and feel impacts our body chemistry. That means everything from stress to pleasure has a profound impact on metabolism.

Think about that for a moment. *Everything that happens in your daily life affects your metabolism!*

When stress hormones get out of whack or stress levels stay chronically elevated over time, they cause a cascade of problems, from wrecking your digestion to causing hormone imbalance and chronic fatigue. I see living proof of this every day in my clients who suffer the effects of stress in their daily lives before doing the Stark Naked 21-Day Metabolic Reset, and there's lots of research proving my point, including studies that show high stress loads can block the production of sex hormones for men and women. As soon as those hormones are out of balance, your metabolism starts falling apart and you will eventually hit the wall from total adrenal burnout. When that happens, you're shot.

Stress is the trigger that breaks homeostasis, the body's ability to maintain internal stability, and affects metabolism. What this means is that you can be eating what some expert deems a "perfect" diet, but if one of your metabolic processes is dysfunctional, your metabolism is going to start to show problems until that dysfunction is fixed. For example, you can eat a low-carb diet, exercise fifteen times a week, and do a thousand crunches a day, but instead of the hard body you're pushing so hard to get, all you're going to end up with is a miserable, frustrating existence.

One of the biggest challenges I face with clients is getting them to believe they aren't being cheated by a faulty metabolism. They are cheating themselves by living the way they do. Oftentimes, clients come to me saying things like, "I can't lose weight because my metabolism is slow," "I don't have the energy," or "Only skinny people have a high metabolism."

I hear the most absurd excuses from people, when in fact it's really a basic metabolic breakdown in their body machinery. Most everyone is born with a healthy metabolism, but, sadly, instead of preserving it, most people will spend their lifetime running it into the ground.

The Metabolic Breakdown Cycle

In the Metabolic Breakdown Cycle, stress, caused by your high-achieving lifestyle, a congested liver, and food-induced inflammation, eventually disrupts hormonal levels, leading to a lethargic metabolism.

METABOLIC BREAKDOWN CYCLE

STRESS (High Achieving Lifestyle, Toxicity, Food-Induced Inflammation) ⇨
Altered Hormones ⇨ Lethargic Metabolism

Physical signs that you are experiencing the Metabolic Breakdown Cycle include low sex drive, intense food cravings, difficulty waking in the morning, low energy throughout the day, gaining fat even though you are eating less and exercising more, sleep issues (exhausted in the morning, can't sleep at night), foggy thinking, increased joint pain, and lack of enjoyment in life.

Your Achilles' heel is the stress hormone known as *cortisol*. Cortisol is a steroid hormone released by the adrenals in response to stress and a low level of blood glucose. Its functions are to increase blood glucose through gluconeogenesis, to suppress the immune system, and to aid the metabolism of fat, protein, and carbohydrates.

Unfortunately, this hormone has gotten a bad rap over the years, but I believe it's misunderstood. Depending on your situation, cortisol can either be your best friend or your worst enemy. We've all heard remarkable stories of superhuman strength in a crisis, such as a woman being able to lift a car off her child with one arm or a man breaking down a door during a fire—that's cortisol working at its finest.

If you ever find yourself being pursued by a lion someday, you better hope your "fight or flight" response is able to fire on all cylinders and release optimal amounts of cortisol to save your life. But too much of this mighty powerful hormone, and it can easily become your worst enemy. Too much cortisol in your system for too long will leave you exhausted, fat, brain-dead, sex deprived, and depressed. As a high achiever, you're probably feeling like this right now. It is the insatiable desire to push physical and mental limits, to create more success in life, and to constantly be better that drives you into a chronic high-stress state. Your body doesn't know the difference between running from a lion or being stuck in traffic—meaning, to your body, stress is stress.

When your body is picking up signs of trouble, it essentially has one way to respond—and that's "fight or flight." Of course, unless you're living in the wilds of East Africa, it is unlikely that you will come across a real lion in your day-to-day activities. As a matter of fact, most likely you will rarely experience the kind of life-or-death situation that our early ancestors relied on the "fight or flight" response to protect them from.

A natural response that developed to help us survive acute bouts of stress is now misfiring within our bodies. As a result of this unnecessary stress response, we are unintentionally being robbed of our health and happiness. Worst of all, it's our own fault. We've created a world of false lions chasing us from the moment we wake to the moment we finally fall asleep—if we fall asleep.

You see, everything you do that causes stress in your life is a lion. The alarm clock startling you out of bed in the morning is a lion. The caffeine in your Starbucks coffee is a lion. Eating a poor breakfast or, worse, skipping breakfast altogether is a lion. Battling traffic is a lion. Dealing with fires at work, managing e-mails, deadlines, negative coworkers, jerk bosses—*all lions.*

Having an argument with your significant other or feeling guilty about missing your child's big game or recital? All these are situations that trigger the same response as a lion chasing you.

Eating what you think is a healthy lunch, not realizing that the almonds and corn you put on your salad may actually be creating large amounts of inflammation (and therefore stress) inside your body—yup, more little lions.

After work you force yourself to hit the gym for your high-intensity workout, because you've read it's the best way to lose your ever-increasing belly fat. What you don't realize is that you've been running from lions all day! By the time you get to the treadmill, you're already completely exhausted, but your body has to dig deeper to find the energy to help you survive yet another bout of stress. You drag your now completely wiped-out self home, grabbing another small cup of coffee-flavored lion on the way.

You force down a bland no-carb dinner, because you've heard that carbs at dinner make you fat. Then you pour yourself a large glass of red lion—oops, I mean wine—to help you unwind and quickly fall asleep on the couch. Your significant other startles you awake and then tells you to come to bed—causing your subconscious to search for the immediate danger. More lions.

As soon as you lie down, he or she starts to get a little frisky, but guess what? Nothing happens on your end, because even if you wanted to, you can't get turned on. You've got no mojo! Great—another lion!

Here's the good news. *It's not your fault your mojo is lacking.*

Your body is inherently wired for survival. When the body thinks it is at high risk, nothing else matters. It wants to keep you alive. There is no way it's going to allow you to get distracted by a possible roll in the hay and end up dead! So you're left lying in bed for the rest of the night, upset and embarrassed, and your now-racing mind is creating more non-life-threatening emotional and mental high-stress situations—releasing more lions. More lions means more cortisol, leading to hormonal disruption, and eventually a lethargic metabolism. It's a vicious and never-ending cycle!

And that is the metabolic breakdown. You will never beat a stress problem by applying more stress.

Eating healthy and exercising are supposed to be fun, simple, and enjoyable. They should be your secret weapons to solve your basic health problems, to help you look great and feel your best. But for too many of my clients—and probably you too—they are two of the most ferocious lions.

When (Seemingly) Good Food Makes You Feel Bad

As a health and wellness expert, I constantly find myself in the unexpected position of having to steer my clients away from eating certain foods that most of us would deem healthy and nutritious, such as blueberries, salmon, broccoli, whole grains, and most nuts. Often, the suspicious culprits are causing digestive intolerances and other disorders that my clients would never have considered were tied to the "healthy" diet they thought they were eating.

Eating healthy and *eating right for your body* are two separate issues. Even if you are eating *healthy* foods, your body may not be metabolizing those foods in a *healthy way*. Inflammation results, causing more stress, bloating, joint pain, water retention, and foggy thinking. Basically, you feel like crap and may not even know it. People learn to live feeling bad. Worse, they accept it as *normal*. It's not normal.

My client Misty was eating all the right foods that were traditionally considered healthy—but for her they were internally raising hell. I remember an e-mail I received from Misty questioning the value of gluten and dairy. Was all of the information she was reading and hearing in the media on the "dangers" of both just hype, or did she really need to be careful? Believe it or not, I commonly get questions from my clients about these, since most nutritionists deem wheat and dairy quite necessary staples in the diet for good health.

Let me regain my composure from that last statement and get the sour taste out of my mouth from having to say it.

Okay. I'm back.

Bull! Neither is necessary!

While following the exact 21-Day Reset outlined in this book, Misty removed all the most common food triggers from her diet, including gluten and dairy, reduced unneeded stressors on the liver, focused on gentle daily liver support, and reduced her exercise. Within 21 days Misty lost 10 pounds and 3 inches off her waist. She no longer needed or craved coffee for energy.

When the time came, I allowed Misty to reintroduce gluten and dairy in the form of pizza after she had had been on the program for 60 days (pizza, mind you, a food that was given to an NFL athlete client of mine during training camp by the team's nutritionist and told it was an amazing source of protein and good carbs!).

Guess what happened?

The retaliation by her body was downright violent. She was extremely fatigued and miserable the following day. She also took multiple unwanted trips to the bathroom. Ouch! Not fun!

Misty had never noticed a reaction to pizza like that before, but definitely recognized the lethargy and depressed feelings from her prior life. She got such great results on the Reset, because she found the source of her Metabolic Breakdown Cycle and fixed it! She was simply eating the wrong foods for her body! Instead of fueling her with great energy, the foods she was eating were really robbing her of her best life and causing serious harm to her metabolism.

I know exactly how Misty felt, because I grew up unaware that an ailment I was suffering from was the result of a reaction to food. I vividly remember being a kid who sucked on four inhalers a day and struggled for every gasp of air; I watched my mom cry because she didn't know what to do to alleviate my struggles to breathe. I spent my early childhood on a dairy farm. I grew up thinking cow's milk was a must and good for strong bones. I consumed an awful lot of dairy, sometimes drinking more than a gallon of milk a week on my own. But milk, as it turned out, was the direct cause of my asthma. Too bad I didn't figure that out until I was thirty-two years old. But once I did, it was amazing how much easier it was to exercise, sleep, and relax, because I was no longer struggling with asthma or being loaded up on the medicine in inhalers.

Just because food is considered healthy and nutritious by someone else's standard, it doesn't mean your body can break it down, assimilate it, or tolerate it in a way that makes it healthy for you.

If you have a digestive disorder or severe food allergy, you already know this. However, if you are unaware of the foods and poor eating habits that might be placing unnecessary stress on your digestive process or causing inflammation, irritation, or other adverse reactions—you could go on feeling bad yet thinking you are eating healthy for years!

Here's what I mean. Are you someone who eats lots of raw veggies thinking they are good for you? Believe it or not, raw vegetables can cause severe bloating and acid reflux. The fructose found in fruits such as mangos, pears, apples, watermelon, grapes, cherries, dried fruits, and fruit juices can cause abdominal pain, bloating, and diarrhea. In some cases, it can even trigger symptoms in patients who suffer from irritable bowel syndrome (IBS) who don't normally have trouble digesting fructose.

Or maybe you're familiar with these habits. Almost all of the clients at Stark are people who are constantly on the go—meaning they are up and out of bed early and often out of the house before the sun rises. By the time most people are rolling out of bed and turning on the morning news, they've been to the gym, showered, and are already at their office or well into their day. For many, breakfast is something they might eat on weekends. This is a huge mistake. We all grew up hearing the line, "Breakfast is the most important meal of the day." And for good reason—it is. You wouldn't head out on a long road trip on an empty tank of gas. Why would you start your day on an empty stomach?

Believe it or not, coffee—even a venti triple latte—*is not a meal!*

But what if you do eat breakfast?

A bowl of Kashi cereal with fat-free milk and a banana may be deemed a healthy breakfast by many, but in reality it's the worst way to start your day! You are far better off eating pure protein such as chicken or bison in the morning than carbs. Why?

Your body is designed to be at its peak energy level between 7:00 and 10:00 A.M. If you don't feed it the right foods to wake your brain up and stabilize energy, you'll be dragging all morning, grumpy, and struggling with hunger. By lunch, you'll be so hungry, you'll more than likely blow it, eating all the wrong foods and sending all of the wrong messages through your system.

On the Stark Naked 21-Day Metabolic Reset, you will learn to eat three perfectly balanced, healthy meals throughout the day for *your* metabolism that will leave you feeling satisfied while stabilizing your blood-sugar levels, which will help level and maintain your mood and energy.

A lot of people supplement their diet by consuming energy drinks instead of eating food. They actually believe these sugar- and caffeine-laden drinks are good for them. Although these drinks might be popular, believe me, they're the devil in disguise. There is nothing in these drinks of any redeeming value. In fact, for many people, the stimulants in these drinks can actually cause problems, such as elevated blood pressure, palpitations, and muscle tremors.

These are all examples of "healthy" foods that may actually be damaging your body and making you feel really bad. So many people never make this connection!

Later in this book you will learn the most common food-sensitivity stressors that are crushing people's metabolisms. We have isolated these over the last two years by looking at labs from hundreds of high achievers just like you. To give you an idea of what I'm talking about, here are some of the other common foods that were causing me problems: salmon, beef, apples, corn, soy, and gluten. These are considered some of the healthiest foods we eat, but consuming these foods was only causing me harm, because my body couldn't break them down and they were, therefore, holding me back from all the promises of eating that healthy diet. It was a real catch-22 until I finally figured it out.

Anyone want to take bets that you're in the same boat?

When you remove the wrong foods for your body from your diet—even if they're thought to be healthy or good for you, these foods are actually acting as toxins in your body—there will be a short-term impact. I've noticed that clients who give up sugar, dairy, wheat, or processed foods go through a period of major discomfort as they purge the toxins from their system. I've even had clients reduce their carbohydrate intake and describe their symptoms a few days later as "flu-like," including a headache, fatigue, achy muscles, and brain fog. What's happening there is the body is making a metabolic switch from burning glucose from carbohydrates for energy to burning fat and protein instead, and that causes those horrible feelings.

So here's the only bad news about doing the Stark Naked 21-Day Metabolic Reset. Depending on your individual state of health and current nutritional strategies, you might have to suffer for a few days before you begin to feel the benefits of the program.

The good news? This transitional period will pass. And once it

does, you will start to feel so good you won't believe you ever allowed yourself to feel that bad.

There's actually a name for this process—the Herxheimer reaction—which is feeling worse before you feel better. Dr. Herxheimer noticed that the symptoms of many patients suffering from syphilis would actually intensify before improving. Interestingly, those patients whose discomfort was the worst during treatment were the strongest and healed the fastest.

Although Dr. Herxheimer's discoveries took place more than a century ago, there is a tremendous amount of relevance to what I see with my clients every day. Anytime you make a radical change in lifestyle, especially when it comes to your diet and health habits, your body will have a strong reaction. From my point of view, the more severe the response, the better the result will be.

Three months into her new lifestyle, Misty sent me an e-mail saying she was down 17 pounds from the start of the program and was superexcited, because she had just returned from purchasing new skinny clothes for summer. She also shared she had been off her antidepressants since we changed her lifestyle and has an amazingly happy outlook on life. The best part of all is that she is experiencing extreme enjoyment being an energetic, present, and naturally happy mom to her children. As for me, receiving these types of e-mails on a regular basis is the best part of my job!

The Downside of Overexercising

Believe it or not, too much of a good thing can actually be destructive and harmful to your health. I see so many of my clients experiencing the downside of overexercising. If you want the greatest benefit of your time in the gym, your recovery has to offset your training volume. If it doesn't, then all of that excessive exercise is only damaging you, not enhancing you. There is a reason the greatest athletes on the

planet sleep 10 to 12 hours per night. They learned early on that their bodies need that much time to rest to enhance recovery from their high volume of physical exercise. Doing this allows them to excel in their field and outperform their competition.

Once you are eating the right foods for your body and your metabolism isn't in a stressed state, it only takes a minimal amount of exercise to get great results.

Don't believe me? Check this out. Most of my professional athlete clients train only 4 days a week for no more than 45 minutes at a time, and they get *insane* results. If you're training more than that and not seeing the kind of results you'd like, I assure you the Metabolic Breakdown Cycle has begun and you need to take steps to fix whatever's broken in your system before you will be happy with your health and fitness results.

Breaking the Cycle

Logically, the solution to solving a stress-driven cycle is not to add more stress to the equation, like a calorie-deprivation plan or more exercise. You can't deprive a high achiever like yourself of carbohydrates, fats, proteins, or calories and expect to perform at an optimal level. You also can't remove yourself from your high-stress, goal-driven world. This will only result in feelings of loss or displacement and depression.

So what is the answer? The ultimate fix for a broken metabolism is to slow down and give your body a break. You must *reset* and *optimize* your metabolism, creating a resiliency that helps you withstand your enemy, *stress.*

Recovery, better known as *rest,* is the one thing you probably don't think you need or make time for, yet it's the one thing science has been showing us makes a major difference in staying healthy and having the stamina to conquer your dreams. Recovery is how

your body recharges itself. It's how it replenishes all your hormones, and it's how your body recovers from the stress you deal with each day. Research has shown that what separates the highest performers in the world from average performers is an increased ability to recover.

In a 2009 study by Eric G. Potterat, in which elite military performers (Navy SEALs) were compared to nonelite military performers, it was discovered that the elite participants demonstrated more substantial heart-rate dipping (the amount of change in heart rate from waking to sleeping) during daily living than the nonelite participants. When these elite performers slept and the parasympathetic nervous system took over to induce recovery, their heart rate dipped by 29 percent versus a 21 percent dip for the nonelite. The greater dip meant they were getting more restorative sleep even when sleep periods were dramatically reduced. We're not all going to be Navy SEALs, but we can all stop focusing on trying to outwork everyone and start focusing more on recovery.

So guess what? From eliminating food-induced inflammation to emphasizing sleep, recovery is the critical component of the Stark Naked 21-Day Metabolic Reset.

Yes, sleep. I figured out that if I can get you to sleep better, you will get better results. Sleep is literally your secret to feeling amazing, looking great, and having the stamina to reach all of your goals in life. It's your greatest ally and the ultimate fountain of youth. Best of all? It's a lot cheaper than Botox and filler!

Still don't believe me? Research from 2007 links greater heart-rate dipping with lower risk of all-cause mortality, and elevated heart rate in general is associated with an increased risk of cardiovascular and noncardiovascular death. That's a scary thought when one of the most common things I see with new clients is an elevated morning resting heart rate.

And if that hasn't convinced you, maybe this will. Cheating your sleep is making you fat!

"Tired" and "fat" seem to go together like peas and carrots, peanut butter and jelly, and pizza and beer. There is no doubt that lack of sleep is related to an increase in hunger and weight gain. Research done by Columbia University looked at eighteen thousand men and women between the ages of thirty-two and fifty-nine and discovered some shocking realities about cheating sleep. Those who slept 4 or less hours a night were 73 percent more likely to be obese than those who slept 7 to 9 hours, and those who slept 5 hours a night were 50 percent more likely to be obese.

If you're not getting enough sleep, your metabolism cannot be supercharged, thereby keeping you lean and healthy.

You're going to hear this a lot throughout this book, but the real secret to great performance in any arena is the ultimate competitive advantage provided by *recovery*. All great performers know this. Have you ever noticed how great performers always share how hard they work, flaunt their crazy exercise regimes, and announce their drive to be the best? What they never share, though, is their game-changing recovery strategies.

Great performers focus on recovery, but they never let their competition know that's their secret. They want them to believe they work insanely hard and never have time to rest. And that's the reason they win, and others don't.

It's Time to Relax and Conquer

When it comes to feeling great, it isn't about working out harder and longer. Feeling great through this method is an empty promise. That old-school approach of using misery, deprivation, and discipline to do whatever it takes to lose weight and look good is over.

Done. As in diddy, diddy, done, done.

It's not about the latest fad diet or calorie count. It's not about overexercising.

Got it?

If you want to really stand out in this world, in your arena, regardless of what it is, then stop stressing your body and overworking and start focusing on the ultimate competitive advantage by learning to *relax and conquer.*

Let's face it. True high achievers won't really slow down or actually take a break until they feel it's critical. And that's exactly why you need this metabolic reset!

You won't slow down or take a break because . . .

You feel "guilty" if you aren't "busy."

You feel "lazy" if you aren't "working."

You feel "useless" if you aren't "doing" something—anything.

Have I hit a nerve yet?

Look, I get it. I work with high achievers every day, and here's what I know for sure. Until you teach high achievers the benefits and the rewards of saving their energy, looking better, getting more done, sleeping better, wanting and having more and better sex, they won't stop—won't take a break and definitely will never see the benefits of resting their body. Trust me, even if you don't know it or aren't willing to admit it yet, these are the things high achievers care about—and rightfully so.

Logically, high achievers need to be supported differently than lazy people who would prefer to never get off of the couch. High achievers need fats, proteins, vegetables, and carbohydrates every day, because they have to manage their stress and replenish that energy they are wiping out day in and day out from their high-stress lifestyle.

The strategies of the Stark Naked 21-Day Metabolic Reset and lifestyle plan are designed to heal the damage caused by the Metabolic Breakdown Cycle and protect your reset metabolism so you don't repeat the cycle over and over again.

Now that you know something's broken, you can choose to fix it.

You can accept feeling awful or choose to feel awesome and full of energy, living your *best* life in good health.

▶ PART TWO

STOP FOOLING YOURSELF AND FIX WHAT'S BROKEN

2

What Do You Mean Stress Is My Problem?

The Impact of High Cortisol Levels

W HAT DO YOU MEAN *stress* is my problem? I don't feel stressed!"

I wish I had a dollar for every time I heard that statement from one of my clients. Even if they are the most stressed-out people on the planet, most of them don't know it!

The majority of us live our complete adult lives dealing with and pushing through symptoms of stress such as anxiety, foggy thinking, bloating, weight and fat gain, lack of sex drive, and sleep issues, just to name a few. According to the Centers for Disease Control (CDC), *up to 90 percent of all illness and disease is stress-related.*

Stop and think about that for a second. How is it possible that my clients aren't aware of their stress?

Because stress isn't always recognizable. In fact, the most dangerous thing about stress, especially for high achievers, is how easily it can creep up on you or, worse, how fast you can learn to accept it as normal.

Ignorance is bliss—except when it comes to stress! When stress is allowed to linger in the body for too long, there's nothing bliss-

ful about it. When you don't know how much stress is really affecting you, you can't possibly understand the toll it's taking. Although
the impact of stress is different for everyone, one thing that's for
sure is that overwhelming stress can and usually does lead to serious health problems, from weakening the immune system, to high
blood pressure, weight gain, sleep loss, lower sex drive, memory loss,
skin conditions, and heart disease. Stress is one of the major causes
of breakdown in the body.

Look, our everyday lives are full of common hassles such as traffic,
deadlines, relationship conflicts, money concerns, child-care issues,
and everyday experiences that can trigger a stress response in the body.
Stress becomes so frequent that you may not recognize the impact it's
having on you. I know it's easy to believe that a little symptom like
being a slow starter in the morning is simply something that comes
with the territory for those with drive and a work ethic, but the truth
is, it's an early sign that stress is negatively impacting your health.

For the majority of my clients, stress is a part of their daily functioning, so much so that they may actually believe they're thriving
because of it.

I have a news flash! They're not. No one really does.

Sure, in small doses, stress can act as a great motivator, but when
it comes in large waves for long periods of time, eventually you will
crash and burn, because your mind and body cannot take the emotional and physical toll.

Stress is a normal physical response to events that make you feel
threatened or upset your balance in some way. When you sense
danger, whether it's real or not, your body's defenses kick into the
"fight or flight" reaction, or what experts often refer to as the stress
response. This response is the body's way of protecting you from danger. If everything is status quo, this response helps you stay focused,
energetic, and alert. However, if you're constantly overwhelmed with
what the body perceives as a threat or problem, you will eventually be
stopped cold in your tracks. Prolonged stress can cause major dam-

Physical Reactions to Stress

Stress impacts everyone differently. Some of the most common symptoms are characteristics of other ailments, so it's easy for most people to brush them off as something else. These "side effects" often include:

- Insomnia
- Clenched or tight jaw
- Teeth grinding at night
- Digestive issues
- Difficulty swallowing
- Tight throat or the feeling of a lump in the throat
- Antsy behavior
- Increased heart rate
- Restlessness
- Achy muscles or muscle tension
- Tight chest or chest pain
- Dizziness or light-headedness
- Hyperventilation
- Sweaty palms
- Nervousness
- Stammering
- High blood pressure
- Low energy
- Fatigue
- Mental slowness
- Negative thoughts
- Constant irritation
- Forgetfulness
- Lack of concentration
- Being easily overwhelmed
- Frustration
- Apathy
- Helplessness
- Low sex drive
- Retreating from friends, family and work (avoidance)

age to your health, mood, body, relationships, and overall quality of life—no matter how great your diet is or how much you exercise.

This chapter is going to take a deeper look at how stress is like an energy vampire that feeds on the body and explore the significant impact it has on us. When you're in a chronic state of stress, it literally robs you of your best self and, therefore, your best health. What if you made some changes and instead of it taking three cups of coffee and a shower to really wake you, you were able to pop right out of bed without an alarm clock and actually enjoy your cup of coffee instead of requiring it for survival? Imagine how much more you could accomplish in your day by waking recharged and ready to conquer the world every morning.

I know most of you believe you handle your stress well, but the likelihood is you probably don't. *Don't wait until things have gotten so bad you need medical intervention to keep you going!*

Over the years, I've met hundreds if not thousands of CEOs and successful businesspeople who have had some type of optimism training. They have been taught to view everything as perfect! Those are the clients that tend to scare me the most.

Why?

Just because you believe your life is stress free, it doesn't mean stress isn't causing damage to your body. For example, stress causes your sex hormones to drop, which means you won't have any sex drive. Your insulin is blunted, causing your blood sugar to skyrocket and your brain to shrink. Your thyroid slows, which means the metabolic pathway for creating energy is disrupted, and the result is total lethargy and unwanted fat gain. These are hardly the traits of a high performer.

A lot of specialists and doctors refer to this condition as "accelerated aging," which is what I was suffering from when I was diagnosed with andropause. Although the idea of accelerated aging may be medically accurate, no one under the age of sixty-five wants to hear that, let alone accept it. I know I didn't!

The accelerated aging process robs you of your quality of life years before you hit rock bottom (more on that in Chapter 6). However, instead of proactively dealing with it, so many people I see in the gym or at one of my seminars choose to ignore it or, worse, glamorize it as one of the traits it takes to truly become successful. I don't want you to be one of those people who hits rock bottom. Once you understand how the stress response works and how it affects your body, you'll be eager to use the 21-Day Reset and get back to your best self.

To understand this better, let's start by exploring what triggers our stress response.

Stress: Your Ultimate Bodyguard

The stress response is triggered by three different categories of stress stimuli. The first category is *life-or-death stress,* which is caused by any situation that threatens your survival, such as almost getting in a car accident or waking at 4:00 A.M. and realizing an intruder is in your house. When life-or-death situations arise, you want to have the necessary energy to respond well. That's why it's important to reduce the drain on your energy reserves from non-life-threatening stress.

The second category is *mental/emotional stress,* which is generated in response to life's challenges and demanding situations. Mental/emotional stress can be caused by life-altering events, such as the death of a loved one, divorce, or the loss of a job, or ordinary events, such as speaking in front of an audience, dealing with a jerk boss, having your spouse yell at you, or simply sitting in traffic. Your mindset determines your response to these types of situations and dictates how your stress response will be activated. With non-life-altering stressors like being stuck in traffic, if you start focusing on negative things that *could* happen, such as being fired for arriving late to a meeting, you will ignite the stress response. Your mind spins with all sorts of terrible possibilities, creating a sense of alarm based on fantasy. In reality, everything is actually okay.

Much of the advice available on how to handle stress deals with this category. If you've read any of it, you know that to prevent your stress response from firing in these non-life-threatening situations, you need to learn how to develop a "bulletproof" mind by curbing your propensity for creating negative outcomes and calming your mind down with activities such as yoga or meditation. In his book *The Way of the SEAL* and online training program *The Unbeatable Mind,* Mark Divine has developed one of my favorite approaches for developing a bulletproof mind.

Even after you've worked hard to build a strong mental outlook, as I have, it's easy for this type of stress to rear its ugly head. A few weeks ago, I was overwhelmed and tired. My wife and I had recently had our third child, so sleep deprivation was causing my mind to play games with me. Tom Ferry, a world famous real-estate coach, walked into the gym at 5:30 A.M. to get a workout in and immediately asked me if I was okay. I don't hide my emotions well. I replied, "Yeah, but my world is out of control. I am feeling so overwhelmed right now."

With a little snicker, he looked around the gym and said, "That's interesting. Your world looks calm and stable to me. You sure it's out of control, or is your thinking making it out of control?"

That simple question brought me back to reality and helped me realize I was creating situations that weren't really happening. It is so easy to let your mind get the best of you and trigger your stress response.

Lifestyle stress is the third category. Reducing lifestyle stress is essential to the Stark Naked 21-Day Metabolic Reset and ultimately will become a part of your everyday lifestyle. Throughout this book you are going to zero in on your most common lifestyle stress triggers and remove them. Lifestyle stress is caused by how you are living your life, your personal behaviors and habits. Cheating sleep, not drinking enough water, eating the wrong foods at the wrong time, and drinking too much coffee are examples of behaviors that trigger the stress response. If you can control these stressors, your life will dramatically change for the better. Let's look at how stress is robbing you of your ultimate energy, focus, and body.

How the Body Responds to Stress

The stress response begins in the brain. When your brain receives signals from your body that something is wrong, it sends an "Oh sh-t" signal to the section of the brain called the hypothalamus. The hypothalamus is a major control center for hormone production, and its primary function is to keep the body in a calm, optimized state. When the hypothalamus receives a stress signal, it works through your nervous system and its crime-fighting partner, the pituitary gland, to heighten your body's ability to respond to danger. The hypothalamus and pituitary trigger your adrenal glands to immediately release the hormone adrenaline followed by the hormone cortisol.

Adrenaline triggers your heart to beat faster, pushing blood to the muscles, heart, and other vital organs. The increase in pulse rate and elevation in blood pressure cause you to start breathing more rapidly and the airways in the lungs to open wide, allowing you to take in extra oxygen that gets carried to the brain, increasing your alertness. Adrenaline also triggers the release of blood sugar (glucose) and fats from storage in the body to help give you the energy to fight or run away from danger. This adrenaline response is so fast, most people don't even realize it's happened; they just know they feel really weird. The adrenals then follow up by releasing the stress hormone cortisol. Cortisol is released to make sure the body stays in this heightened state for as long as it takes to deal with the threat. Once the threat has subsided, cortisol levels decrease, allowing the body to go into recovery mode and replenish itself for the next life-or-death situation.

Your Inner Hulk, or When Stress Becomes Your Evil Foe

The transformation of Bruce Banner into the Hulk in the movie *The Incredible Hulk* is an excellent example of the stress response in action—and how it can become your worst enemy. A quiet child, Bruce Banner grew up in a very stressful environment. He lived with an abusive father and was constantly picked on by school bullies. Extremely intelligent, he eventually became a nuclear engineer for the military. During a test of a bomb he created, Banner was exposed to high levels of gamma radiation, transforming him into the Hulk. Because Banner had such a stressful childhood, his stress response system was very sensitive, and as soon as his body released the stress hormone adrenaline, the brutish Hulk would emerge.

Like all of us, the Hulk does not respond well to stress. He has a childlike intelligence, makes poor decisions, and becomes a very destructive menace to society. Sound anything like how you respond when stressed? Every once in a while the Hulk would do something heroic, but just like our own typical responses under stress, those times are few and far apart. Banner eventually discovered strategies to manage his response to stress, so that the Hulk would only emerge under extreme situations, not at the drop of a hat.

We all have a Hulk inside of us. It can be used for the greater good in extreme situations, but most of us have yet to obtain control of our inner Hulk. Your inner Hulk emerges most frequently from mental/emotional triggers, like sitting in traffic. I love watching the Hulk appear in cars around me in Southern California traffic. The inner Hulk causes people to honk and scream, slam

---

Chef Amar Santana, owner of Broadway by Amar Santana
Laguna Beach, California
Age thirty-two

▶ *Chef Amar Santana is one of Orange County's rising stars in the culinary world with his wildly successful flagship restaurant Broadway by Amar Santana in Laguna Beach. A chef's lifestyle is a big ball of stress. Their days start early and end late! Good luck getting them to eat a healthy diet, let alone find time to exercise.*

Amar's life was no different when he came to me looking for help. He had put on 50 pounds over the prior year and developed horrible sleep habits. His diet consisted of eating one calorie-laden meal at night, and most of his sleep came during a 2-hour nap he snuck in at some point each day. He was only thirty-two years old, but he looked much older because he was exhausted. On top of that, Amar felt overwhelmed and was tired of being overweight.

Although Amar has had success in the past with exercise pro-

their steering wheels, and drop not just F bombs, but A–Z bombs.

You definitely want your inner Hulk to emerge in life-or-death situations, but having your inner Hulk appear during a traffic jam or from drinking too much coffee is far from beneficial for you. It is actually very damaging. When cortisol is chronically elevated, your body is stuck in the revved-up fight-or-flight response all the time— which may sound good, but the impact is actually horrible. That would be like trying to reach 90 miles per hour on the highway with your car in first gear! Worse, a lot of people are stuck in that mode trying to sleep at night. Good luck with that!

High achievers are prone to abusing the fight-or-flight response, because they get used to living in this heightened Hulk state and consider it a "normal" way of life. They are experts at ignoring stress signals and have absolutely no idea that their stress response has

---

grams and extreme diets, he had never committed to making a change in his lifestyle. As with most programs, if you don't make a lifestyle change, the weight comes right back, and the stress from the extreme dieting and exercise actually contribute to more fatigue once the program is stopped.

After completing the Stark Naked 21-Day Metabolic Reset, Amar lost 14 pounds, which was a fantastic jump-start to his weight loss program and the incentive he needed to help him stick with it. The best part? He was able to fall asleep at night without relying on alcohol, and his sleep was uninterrupted through the night. Also because he no longer needed the 2-hour nap each day, he had plenty of time to add exercise back into his lifestyle.

Today Amar's life is still crazy stressful, but once we reset his metabolism, we were able to build resiliency to stress into his routine. He sleeps, which is critical, he stabilizes his blood sugar by eating the right foods at the right times throughout the day, and he is no longer dehydrated.

kicked in. I hate to break it to you, but although you may believe you're superhuman, just as my kids do when they put on their super-hero costumes, you are not. When you run around like the Hulk for too long, your stress-response system begins to falter from over-work, causing the Metabolic Breakdown Cycle to start, leaving you exhausted and feeling bad all the time.

There is a price to pay every time your stress response is turned on.

Stress and the Metabolic Breakdown Cycle

As we learned earlier, cortisol elevation in acute life-or-death bouts is awesome, but when it's left stuck in the "on" position 24/7, it creates problems. When you are stuck in a heightened state, you will actually feel invigorated and alive. It's called an adrenaline rush, and you feel as though you are conquering life, but as it stays on, you slowly become "tired but wired" and eventually become downright exhausted. That's The Metabolic Breakdown Cycle at work.

Let's look at this a little closer. Chronic cortisol release has a negative effect on all other hormones. Remember that the body is built first and foremost to survive at all costs. This means your body will do whatever it takes to survive right now! It doesn't care that the actions it takes will lead to a heart attack in five years. It only cares about surviving *now.* When you live in a constant state of stress, the body is continuously being forced to take action for your immediate survival. Unfortunately, this is at the expense of all other metabolic systems.

Chronic cortisol elevation affects your body in numerous ways, but for our purposes I am going to focus on what I feel are the "Big Four," meaning the effects that have the greatest impact on you: elevated blood sugar, suppressed sex hormones, an underactive thyroid, and extra belly fat. When your body is exposed to long-term elevated cortisol, these Big Four will leave you fat, sluggish, uninterested in sex, and far from your intellectual peak.

Cortisol and Blood Sugar

When cortisol is elevated, the body upregulates glucose and fats for instant energy, but blunts the effect of insulin, essentially rendering cells insulin-resistant. Not only are blood-glucose levels high, but insulin is unable to perform its regular function of maintaining normal glucose levels. This puts extra stress on the pancreas, as it continues to produce increasing amounts of insulin in response to high glucose levels.

If cortisol is elevated 24/7, your blood sugar will also stay elevated. Long-term elevated blood sugar has been shown to negatively affect our brains, actually taking away from our intelligence. Research has linked elevated blood sugar to a reduction in the size of the hippocampus, the part of the brain responsible for memory. In his book *Why Isn't My Brain Working?*, Dr. Datis Kharrazian shows that millions of Americans are affected by brain damage caused by blood-sugar imbalances.

Elevated blood-sugar levels also increase fat levels, because muscle cells are not allowed to accept the glucose into the cell due to the dampened insulin response. Eventually the liver has to do something with the excess buildup of glucose in the bloodstream, so it recycles it as fatty acids and shuttles it off to be stored as fat.

So many people believe that you have to overconsume carbohydrates to create blood-sugar issues, but to validate my point that blood sugar can become an issue due to stress alone, I have even seen the impact of high cortisol levels on blood sugar in high-level athletes, especially top-level CrossFit athletes, who avoid carbs like the plague. They haven't had a carb in five years, yet they are prediabetic. Controlling cortisol is critical for long-term blood-sugar management.

Cortisol and Sex Hormones

Did you know stress can suppress your sex hormones? Yes, you read that right. Stress and sex don't mix. In men, elevated cortisol levels reduce the production of testosterone, an essential component for a healthy sex drive. In women, it causes a cascade of hormonal imbalances resulting in low libido. Low sex-hormone levels can rob you of your sex drive, take away your overall zest for life, and even lead to an early death.

Prolonged cortisol elevations also decrease the liver's ability to clear excess estrogens from the blood, leading to estrogen dominance and accumulation of fat on the hips, thighs, back of the arms, and chest. This estrogen buildup also has a negative effect on the thyroid, which I'll explain next. You have to get your cortisol under control if you want your sex hormones optimized. In Chapter 5, we'll explore in more detail how stress robs your mojo (yes, a whole chapter on mojo!), but for now the crucial point is this: when cortisol levels are elevated, sex-hormone production is slowed.

Cortisol and the Thyroid

Chronic stress and elevated cortisol levels wreak havoc on your thyroid in a number of ways. A proper amount of cortisol is very important for normal thyroid function. Cortisol works in a synergistic fashion with the thyroid hormone at the cellular level, making the thyroid hormone work more efficiently. When cortisol levels are too high, the brain will reduce the body's ability to make more thyroid hormone, which over time results in sluggishness, extreme fatigue, and other symptoms of hypothyroidism. Basically, your body is too busy focusing all its energy on keeping your inner Hulk amped up to maintain proper thyroid function, leading you to the extreme consequence of the Metabolic Breakdown Cycle.

Last, as mentioned in the previous section, when cortisol levels are elevated, so are estrogen levels. High levels of estrogen interrupt thyroid function by increasing levels of the thyroid-binding protein thyroxine-binding globulin (TBG). Thyroid hormones are bound to this protein and inactive while they travel through your body in the blood. Once they reach your cells, they become unbound and active to do their work. If there is too much TBG, thyroid hormones remain bound, unable to get into cells and therefore unable to do their work. Hypothyroid symptoms are the result.

Cortisol and Belly Fat

Cortisol has the ability to trigger fat loss and fat storage. For example, cortisol triggers fat release during controlled periods of exercise, as long as you don't eat carbohydrates prior to the exercise. But when cortisol is chronically elevated, it promotes the storage of fat and relocates excess circulating fat to your abdomen. If left unchecked, this results in weight gain and a resistance to weight loss. It gets even worse when insulin joins the party.

Insulin activity shuts down the fat-releasing activity of other hormones like cortisol, and when these two are partying together, they trigger the release of the major fat-storage enzyme lipoprotein lipase. Hello, belly fat. Welcome to the cortisol and insulin fiesta. Olé!

In addition, consistently high blood-glucose levels and blunted signaling of insulin leads to cells that are starved of glucose. But those cells are crying out for energy. This causes your appetite to fire, leading to overeating, as your body compels you to replenish for the next time your life is at risk. This is when we usually start devouring all our comfort foods, like ice cream, that combine fat and sugar. And, of course, unused glucose is eventually converted to fatty acids by the liver and stored as body fat, primarily around the belly.

Adding Insult to Injury

Wow! We are on a cortisol roll. We have covered the Big Four negative impacts on your body caused by elevated cortisol levels, so let's just add a little insult to injury.

Not only does stress destroy how we feel, look, and perform; it's also a key player in increasing our risk of disease and early death. Hypertension (high blood pressure), hyperlipidemia (elevated lipids), and hyperglycemia (elevated glucose) have all been linked to elevated cortisol levels. Individuals with a high waist-to-hip ratio (which identifies visceral obesity, excessive fat accumulation around the organs within the abdominal cavity) are at a greater risk for developing cardiovascular disease, type 2 diabetes mellitus, and cerebrovascular disease.

As you can see, stress destroys your ability to live optimally. Do you understand now how vital it is for you to wrap a lasso around your cortisol and get it under control?

Mike, SWAT team member
California
Age forty

▶ When I first met Mike as a potential client, I immediately knew our biggest struggle was going to be working around his insane sleep schedule. The first day we met, he had been so busy with SWAT calls, he had only averaged around 3 hours of sleep a night over the prior 72 hours. Combine that with the constant stress of raiding houses of dangerous criminals, uncertain of what's waiting for him on the other side of the door each time, and he had the perfect storm for an extremely stressful lifestyle.

Mike had been a collegiate fullback. When we met, one of his primary goals was to get his college body back before turning the big four-oh. He had three months to make it happen. His starting weight was 225 pounds, which was promising, but his body fat of 18.2 percent was far from ideal. Mike wanted to keep his weight above 210, but get his body fat back to 10 percent. He also wanted more energy to train harder, which Mike knew was

How the Stark Naked 21-Day Metabolic Reset and Lifestyle Control Your Inner Hulk

All three categories of stress can trigger your inner Hulk when not managed appropriately, but the main culprits are the category-three lifestyle stressors. You're probably not even aware of them. Imagine if Bruce Banner knew that cow's milk triggered the Hulk to emerge. Would he drink it every day? No way, but we do silly things like this each day. Now I am not saying that cow's milk is a trigger for everyone, but you would be amazed at the number of people it does affect.

Reducing poor lifestyle choices that trigger category-three stressors is the foundation of the Stark Naked 21-Day Metabolic Reset

---

lacking because he was forcing himself to go to the gym every morning instead of being excited about working out.

Oh, how I love a good challenge!

Since I knew Mike's work schedule wasn't going to change, I immediately put him on the Stark Naked 21-Day Metabolic Reset, so I could quickly fix what was broken inside Mike's body and establish a healthy foundation to create a resiliency to the stress of Mike's work and lifestyle. I wanted Mike to reach his goal instead of continuing his frustrating cycle of constantly fighting himself and getting nowhere despite trying.

After the initial 21-day phase, Mike's weight dropped to 221 pounds and his body fat to 14 percent. He lost 10 pounds of fat and added 6 pounds of lean muscle mass just by resetting his metabolism and allowing his body to recover from his extreme stress. Today at forty years old Mike weighs 215 pounds with a body fat of 10 percent and holding! His energy is through the roof, his training in the gym has gone to a whole new level, and, as he puts it, "I haven't felt this good since I was in my early twenties." I call that a win for both of us!

and lifestyle. Throughout this book you are going to zero in on the three most common triggers—a stressful lifestyle, toxicity, and food sensitivities—remove them, and learn to calm your inner Hulk. I've taken all of the guesswork out of it for you. This program corrects the poor lifestyle decisions triggering your stress response. Just follow the program exactly as laid out, and you can rest assured that the multiple Hulk triggers robbing you of your best self are being removed. If you skip any of the strategies to reset your metabolism in Chapter 11, you are allowing a Hulk trigger to run free and prevent your metabolism from a full reset. It's only 21 days!

Give your inner Hulk a break! Your health, energy, waistline, sex drive, and those around you will thank you.

Make a commitment to take control of your lifestyle and apply the given strategies in this book to support your liver, remove food-driven inflammation, enhance your sleep, balance your daily or weekly exercise and recovery, and feed your high-performing lifestyle in a new way, so your inner Hulk only appears when you really need it!

Reducing the lifestyle stressors that trigger your inner Hulk is the key to resetting your metabolism.

The eleven fundamentals of the Stark Naked 21-Day Metabolic Reset in Chapter 11 (see page 204) remove the multiple Hulk triggers robbing you of your best self. The first four are specifically designed to reduce your stress load and help you get better control of your cortisol.

1. Hydrate.
2. Sleep 7 to 9 hours a night every night.
3. Drastically reduce your intense exercise.
4. Commit to daily acts of relaxation.

Your Liver Needs Some Love

The Impact of Toxicity on the Body

WHETHER YOU REALIZE IT OR NOT, we live in a really toxic world. When I speak of toxins, I don't mean just pesticides or hazardous waste. What I am referring to is anything, whether a chemical or poison, that is known to have a harmful effect on the body. There are currently over eighty thousand known chemicals in our daily environment. Fifteen thousand of these are used in high volumes in the United States. Today, the United States produces over 300 billion pounds of chemicals a year. The average American is directly exposed to over 1,500 pounds of these chemicals annually, many of which are known carcinogens, substances directly involved in causing cancer.

That's a lot of dangerous chemicals to be swimming in! When asked, most people are unable to name one single toxic chemical that is a known health risk, and yet they live among thousands of them every day. As a society, we tend to have an awful lot of faith that big industry has our ultimate safety in mind over their own profits when it comes to creating and marketing the products they sell us.

What's even more frightening to me is the number of toxins our children are exposed to—even before they are born. This concerns me so much, because I have three beautiful children whose blood-brain barrier won't be fully developed until around the age of twenty, leaving their brains unprotected from these chemicals. It's scary to think that my little boy Gavin, born in October 2014, was exposed to hundreds of different toxins before he was even born.

Research presented by the Environmental Working Group shows there could have been as many as 287 different chemicals passing through the umbilical cord directly into the placenta. Of these, 217 are known neurotoxins, poisons that affect the brain and nervous system, and 180 are ones that we know cause cancer in humans and animals. The reported chemicals are coming from herbicides, household products, consumer products, stain and oil repellant used in fast-food packaging, flame retardants, and pesticides.

Even though my wife took great care of herself throughout her pregnancy, it would be virtually impossible for her to avoid these toxins. They're everywhere and enter the body through the food you eat, the air you breathe, the water you drink (especially from that pretty and convenient plastic bottle), the clothes you wear, the products you use to clean your home, the cell phone you're talking on, and the lotions and balms you lather all over your skin every day thinking you're caring for your body, when you are actually wreaking havoc on it by adding to the toxicity.

What's the result of all of this exposure? Unfortunately, our bodies have become a toxic dumping ground, and we are paying a massive price for it.

Once our bodies have been exposed to these harmful toxins, they are processed through the liver and kidneys. Whenever possible, our body eliminates them in the form of sweat, breath, urine, and feces. Toxins not eliminated are retained. Because toxins are so damaging, the Stark Naked 21-Day Metabolic Reset is designed to help you cleanse the toxins from your system and relieve the stress you've unknowingly been placing on your body over the years, or as I like to call it, "love your liver," every day.

If you're the grumpy morning person everyone avoids talking to before 10:00 A.M., the person who needs to hit the snooze button on your alarm multiple times, stealing every last possible minute of sleep before getting out of bed, someone who needs a couple of cups of coffee to calm the beast and wake up before you can function in the world, then you are *definitely* someone who will benefit from loving on your liver. (Naturally, your kidneys are part of the detoxification process as well and will be supported in this process, but in an effort to keep things supersimple I've chosen to focus on the big driver of detoxification, your liver.)

How do you accomplish this?

First, eliminate the toxins you are eating and drinking. Without realizing it, most people eat and drink so many toxic substances, thinking they aren't causing any additional stress on the body, contributing to the onset or flare-up of a disease, or creating complications for themselves—but they are.

For example, caffeine is a favorite vice among my clients. But it's also one of the most taxing stressors on your liver and adrenal glands. One report I read from the Department of Molecular and Cell Biology at the University of California, Berkeley, stated there are up to one thousand chemicals in a single cup of coffee.

Alcohol is another major culprit. Aside from the hangovers, headaches, and other occasional unpleasant side effects, drinking alcohol depletes nutrients, especially B vitamins that are needed for metabolism and . . . what was that darn word I was looking for?

Oh yes, *memory*!

That's what causes the occasional forgetfulness about what went on the night before! Worse, breaking down alcohol exhausts your liver, making it harder to eliminate the unwanted poisons from your body. Not to mention that too much alcohol can damage or destroy liver cells. That's not to say you should never drink alcohol—you can.

Like everything, moderation and drinking some green tea before a night out on the town will help your liver function a little more effectively. Staying superhydrated is always a good idea too!

And finally, there's sugar. Kicking the sugar habit is hard, but it's so worth it. If I can get clients off sugar for 21 days, they rarely go back. It's akin to any drug detox program out there, because sugar is as addictive as most drugs. Think about it. Eating anything with refined sugar only makes you want to eat more. The brain depends on blood glucose for its energy. Eating sucrose can cause a plethora of problems, especially when it comes to blood-glucose levels.

Remember that famous trial where the attorney used the Twinkie defense, claiming his client's irrational behavior was impacted by his high-sugar junk-food diet? Although I am not sure I believe Twinkies will cause you to do crazy things, I do know this: There's no real nutritional value in eating one!

If you want to get off the sugar train once and for all, you have to start by cutting down or eliminating all refined sugars from your diet.

Guess what?

Refined sugar is hiding in the most unexpected places, such as those "healthy" juice drinks you think are good for you, your favorite marinara sauce, and every meal replacement bar! Read the labels on some of your favorite so-called healthy foods sometime and I'll bet you'll be shocked by the amount of sugar you'll discover among those ingredients. Eliminating sugar isn't easy, but once you kick the habit, food will start to taste better, and you will start to feel better too.

Now, I want to be up front and tell you the Stark Naked 21-Day Metabolic Reset is not an extreme detoxification program. If it were, you'd probably quit before seeing the kind of results you're looking for.

How do I know?

Like so many of my clients, I have punished myself over the years by trying many different extreme detox protocols. In fact, I was obsessed with wanting to understand them, because clients would come to me asking about them or after doing one. Most often, their results were consistently negative. Curious and perplexed, I didn't know the reason why, but I wanted to find out so I could help right the wrong.

Sure, they lost weight, but their body fat didn't change or, worse, it actually got higher. That meant they just stripped off muscle instead of fat, which is never desirable. In my mind, a detox should only be done if it will improve one's health, not worsen it. Although a detox cleanse may indeed help you shed a few pounds, it's likely that the lost weight is primarily water, which will come right back on as soon as you veer off the plan—even the slightest bit. This only leads to frustration and setbacks.

So how can you see effective results from a detox?

I have seen great success with my clients by simply removing any unnecessary sources of daily liver burden, so the liver can focus on the backed-up toxic junk that has been stored in your fat. Doing this enhances the liver's ability to work more efficiently with less effort. The body is designed to constantly filter toxins we ingest. If we can aid in that process, we will feel and look better.

What does this mean for you? Sorry to say—okay, not *that* sorry to say—that it means you will have to go without coffee, alcohol, and sugar for 21 days. But guess what? It's only for 21 days!

Give yourself 21 days, and you will experience the ultimate benefit: enhanced fat burning.

Yep, you read that right!

When the liver can catch up on the work it has fallen behind on, better fat metabolism is the outcome. After the 21-day Reset, if you still feel you want to include these toxins in your diet, I will teach you how to strategically reintroduce each of them without undoing all of the progress you've made.

A Healthy Liver

Your liver is the second-largest organ in your body (your skin is the largest). The liver is extremely valuable to the human body. It is responsible for over six hundred metabolic activities and actually has the ability to regenerate after being damaged.

Your liver is designed to survive at all costs. When your liver is overwhelmed, it goes into major survival mode. It will focus less on making sure your metabolism is firing on all cylinders and more on protection. It will start storing as fat the toxins it can't process and clear immediately.

How does this impact you? I don't care how much you control your calories and kill yourself on the treadmill, if your liver is over-whelmed, you are stuck in neutral—meaning that even if you're doing all the right things, you will never meaningfully move the needle on the scale.

If you want to get the most out of the Stark Naked 21-Day Metabolic Reset, it's important to understand the major role your liver plays in your everyday life. Most people know they have a liver, but few understand its function and purpose, so let's break it down to help you understand why a healthy liver is essential to your health and ultimately your success.

A healthy liver:

Cleans toxins and wastes from your blood. It polices your blood looking for toxins that are a dangerous threat to your body. When a toxin tries to sneak in, the liver ambushes the threat, cuffs it, and escorts it out of the body via pathways like sweat, breath, urine, and feces. This is a good thing, or like my daddy used to say, "Don't let the door hit you where the good Lord split you!"

Looks for the VIP citizens known as vitamins and minerals. It processes these highly valuable assets and prepares them, so your body can use them to work properly. Vitamins and minerals are used for things like enhancing your immune system, aiding in digestion, producing energy, protecting your cells from damage during stress and exposure to toxins, protecting your body from viruses and bacteria, and building strong bones and teeth.

Plays an important role in digestion. It is the central hub for metabolizing all calories and is responsible for processing proteins, fats, and carbohydrates. It is involved in protein synthesis, processing amino acids from broken-down protein so the body can use them. The liver makes a greenish-yellow gooey substance called bile, which is stored in the gallbladder. This substance is critical for the digestion and absorption of fats. The liver is also responsible for aiding in the management of blood sugar. The liver can store excess glucose in the blood as glycogen to be used in times of low blood sugar or other emergency energy needs. A healthy liver processes proteins, fats, and carbohydrates efficiently, allowing you to enjoy the benefits of better energy, low body fat, and a sharp mind.

Makes cholesterol. Relax! Cholesterol is a good thing. It's the backbone of your sex hormones. It also makes the base proteins needed for blood clotting.

Metabolizes steroidal hormones, such as the sex hormones and aldosterone (controls the balance of sodium, potassium, and water in your body), once they are done doing their job in the body. You will learn more about the liver and sex hormones later in this chapter and in Chapter 5, but they essentially control your sex drive. When the liver efficiently breaks down aldosterone, water retention is under control and you're able to keep your blood pressure in check. It can also slow down those pesky bathroom trips during the night.

An Unhealthy Liver

Now, that's what happens in a beautiful, optimally functioning liver—something few of us have. In reality, that is far from how most people's normal livers function these days. Many of my clients will try to defend themselves and their livers by showing me their "excellent" liver enzyme levels on recent blood work. However, I am usually the bearer of bad news when I have to explain they're not off the hook, because their liver is still suffering and causing them major problems.

How do I know? At Stark, we run a simple urine lab test called the Urinary Bile Acid Sulfates (UBAS), which looks at liver function efficiency by testing its role as a filter of bile acids. Bile acids are a normal component of blood that your liver is responsible for clearing out. If you have a sluggish or overwhelmed liver, bile acids build up in your blood, forcing the kidneys to convert them to sulfates and excrete them through your urine. When sulfates are present at high levels in the urine, it's a clear sign your liver is working overtime and not keeping up with its workload.

Here's the scary part. Every person we ran this test on had elevated UBAS levels, yet the majority of those people had normal liver enzyme labs. What this tells us is a normal liver enzyme result doesn't necessarily mean you're safe.

If you have never had a UBAS test but have normal liver enzyme levels and are wondering if your liver is having an effect on your health, your cholesterol profile can give you a pretty good idea. The majority of your total cholesterol is produced in your liver. When your liver starts to get bogged down by stress, toxins, and too much sugar and fat consumption, cholesterol production can be thrown off balance. One of the liver's jobs is to use low-density lipoprotein (LDL) cholesterol to stimulate bile-salt production to help deal with fats in the blood. When fats in the blood begin to accumulate because of a sluggish liver, the need for LDL cholesterol and bile salt increases. An elevation in LDL cholesterol and triglycerides (a marker of how much fat is in the blood) is a sign that your liver is in overdrive. Your liver is not efficiently burning fat and is more than likely clogged up and tilted toward storing fat instead of metabolizing it.

Now that I have your attention, let's explore how your sluggish liver may be affecting your energy, weight, and mojo.

Sluggish Liver, Low Energy, Weight Gain, Low Mojo

A sluggish liver will have a dramatic effect on your energy. Toxins build up in the blood, reducing its capacity to carry oxygen and nutrients required for energy production. The result is constant fatigue. It can also have a negative effect on your energy by slowing down your thyroid.

The thyroid needs the liver to activate its hormone, so the body can actually use it. When activation is slowed, the thyroid struggles to do its job. When that happens, your metabolism is forced to slow down, and fatigue results.

As far as weight gain goes, a sluggish liver is forced to store fat instead of burn it, leaving you with a nice buildup of fat, especially around your belly. It's tough enough to exercise when your liver is storing fat and your circulation is poor, but combine that with a slow metabolism that prevents your thyroid from optimally burning energy during exercise, and it's next to impossible to lose weight. This is what causes most people to just give up on their weight-loss goals.

Finally, a sluggish liver is causing your sex hormones to go haywire. The liver is responsible for the elimination of excess estrogens. When the liver is backed up, this process is slowed and estrogens begin to build in the body, causing an imbalance. Women, this creates all kinds of havoc in your world. The buildup of estrogen can cause symptoms such as insomnia, fat accumulation around the hips and thighs, mood swings, foggy thinking, enhanced PMS symptoms, water retention, hair loss, and headaches.

Men, this buildup of estrogen can interfere with your fertility (impotence), sexual function (low sex drive and erectile dysfunction), and put you at risk for circulatory problems, heart attack, and stroke. Not to mention fat accumulation around your chest (yup, moobs, or man boobs) and thighs, thinning of your body hair, and depression. No fun if you're a guy who wants to maintain his manliness!

At Stark we track and monitor everything monthly to make sure people are making positive progress. If they aren't, we can make quick adjustments, so people aren't wasting time or effort. One month we noticed that my business partner Todd's body fat had gone up out of the blue. Worse, his skin folds in the estrogen areas started creeping up too. He was laying down fat on his chest and especially his thighs. We refer to that as "feminizing" at Stark. He swore up and down he was following the protocols we designed and was blaming my team for feminizing him.

We dug real deep and discovered he had switched his body wash and lotion recently to products that were packed full of estrogen-mimicking parabens, and they were taking a toll on Todd's manhood. We had him go back to his old body wash and lotion and gave him some extra liver support for 30 days, and his body returned to his nonfeminized masculine body, or at least what he thinks is his masculine body.

Now do you believe me when I say it's worth your time and effort to support your liver?

The Impact of Chemical Toxins on Your Liver

In his book *Achieving Victory Over a Toxic World,* Dr. Mark Schauss writes that in retaliation against the toxic burden, the body will store toxins in fat and actually turn down the internal temperature to help

Signs and Symptoms of a Sluggish Liver

- Elevated LDL cholesterol
- Low HDL cholesterol
- Elevated triglycerides
- Expanding waistline
- Weight gain on the hips and thighs
- Abdominal bloating
- Inability to digest fatty foods
- Loss of appetite, especially in the morning
- Skin issues like psoriasis, eczema, acne, rashes, and itchy skin
- Low energy especially in the morning and after meals
- Unstable blood sugar
- Dizziness
- Sleep disturbances
- Moodiness
- Depression
- Hot flashes
- Irregular periods
- Intolerance to alcohol
- Intolerance to caffeine
- Swollen feet
- Swollen abdomen
- Bad breath
- Dark urine or stool
- Easy bruising
- Body odor
- Sensitivities to smells from perfumes, chemicals, paints, and cleaners

keep these toxins at bay. This slight drop in body temperature slows the resting metabolic rate enough to cause unwanted weight gain. If you've ever attempted an extreme approach to weight loss, you have probably experienced the wrath of all the toxins being released in the bloodstream too fast from the fat, eventually making you sick.

Eating a clean diet and limiting your caffeine, alcohol, and sugar intake will take some pressure off your liver, but there are so many more toxins that you're being exposed to on a daily basis that are causing health problems for you. Environmental pollutants burden you as well. But the toxins I've seen that cause the most trouble are found in the solvents used to make cleaning and personal-care products, the products you are choosing to put in your environment and even rub into your skin. Before you slather on your favorite body lotion, I want you to turn the bottle around and read the ingredients. Ask yourself this one simple question: *Do I know what all these chemicals are?* If your answer is no, why in the world are you putting it on your skin?

According to the Federal Food, Drug, and Cosmetic (FD&C) Act, cosmetics are defined by their intended use as "articles intended to be rubbed, poured, sprinkled or sprayed on, introduced into, or otherwise applied to the human body . . . for cleansing, beautifying, promoting attractiveness, or altering the appearance." Under the FD&C Act, cosmetics and their ingredients are not required to undergo approval before they are sold to the public. This includes skin moisturizers, perfumes, lipsticks, nail polish, mascara, facial makeup, shampoos, hair coloring, toothpastes, and deodorants.

I have even found scientifically proven dangerous chemicals in products for babies. Parabens, for example, have been shown to be an estrogen-mimicking chemical in rats and the methyl form has been found in the cells of breast-cancer tissue. I found methyl parabens in an old bottle of baby bedtime lotion. When my daughter was a baby, I had rubbed this on her after her baths, thinking I was being a loving father. I also remember my wife complaining about my holding my daughter when I had cologne on, because it made her smell like a man. Imagine my guilt when I researched the safety of colognes and found that my cologne at that time was rated as the most dangerous.

The average woman puts three to five hundred chemicals on her skin before leaving the house every morning. The typical perfume has over two hundred different chemicals alone! As a result of all of that primping, your liver is bombarded with toxins and angry at you before 8:00 A.M.! And the only person you can blame is yourself! Ouch!

Generally, the Food and Drug Administration (FDA) regulates these products after they have been released into the marketplace. There is no preapproval system in place except for color additives, such as those found in self-tanners. This means that manufacturers may use any ingredient or raw material in a product and sell it without a government review or approval. Parabens, for example, are used as a preservative and aren't just found in baby products. It is estimated that they are present in 75 to 90 percent of all beauty products. The parabens and chemicals in these products are being linked to issues like hormone disruption, infertility, cancer, headaches, skin irritants, allergies, and liver and kidney damage, to name a few.

Phthalates are another scary family of chemicals that are usually hidden on labels. These are typically hidden in the word "fragrance" on most products that have a smell and in nail polish. Phthalates have been shown to also be an estrogen mimicker and are linked to cancer and liver damage. The European Union has completely banned dibutyl phthalate (DBP) from cosmetics and baby products. That's scary. What do they know? What are we turning a blind eye to?

The list of "at risk" chemicals in solvents is constantly growing. It's time to wake up to the reality that solvents could be a major source of toxic overload for you and may be causing you some serious issues. It's my opinion that smelling great isn't worth losing my testosterone over. Wow. That brings back serious memories of a young man in my middle school who wore so much Polo cologne, he literally had a green cloud floating above him. Makes you cringe even more now, doesn't it?

Most of us apply somewhere in the neighborhood of 126 unique ingredients to our skin daily without giving any of them a second thought. But we should, because chemicals from all of our coveted beauty products don't pass through the digestive system, where they might be filtered. Instead, they head right into your bloodstream and therefore can be extremely toxic and quite dangerous to your health. According to the Environmental Working Group, one out of every 120 products on the market contains ingredients certified by government authorities as *known or probable human carcinogens*. One out of every 13 women and one out of every 23 men—12.2 million adults—are exposed to ingredients that are known or probable carcinogens every day through their use of personal-care products.

The regulatory requirements governing the sale of cosmetics are not as stringent as those that apply to other FDA-regulated products. In fact, cosmetics and toiletries are some of the least regulated and scrutinized products available. Although companies are not required to substantiate performance claims or conduct safety testing, if safety has not been substantiated, the product's label must read "WARNING: The safety of this product has not been determined."

Most people falsely believe that if a product is on the shelf, it can't be harmful. Of course, we all know that's not true. Cigarettes are a great example of that.

But hardly anyone thinks of perfume or body lotion in that same category. And really, why would you? Companies are required to list all the ingredients in order of use, but they are not required to test their products for safety, so no one understands the risk of using those products they believe are good for them. To be fair, that doesn't mean that all cosmetic companies don't have safety standards, but it does mean that many such claims as "natural," "botanical," and "organic" are useless. The FDA can take action against a product only if it has enough scientific proof that the product is actually dangerous.

Do yourself a favor and take some time to research all the products in your medicine cabinet or bathroom to see what toxins you are using on your skin or hair, brushing your teeth with, breathing in, or ingesting on a daily basis. If you can pronounce the ingredients or know what they are, it's a good bet the product is probably safe. Any ingredient that has too many syllables or is unrecognizable is most likely a chemical or toxin. Remove the dangerous products from your shelves. Your liver will thank you and, believe me, you will notice a significant difference in how you look and feel.

I have seen enough improvement in people who have removed questionable solvents that I now am down to using only two products: Dr. Bronner's Castile Liquid Soap and Jungleman all-natural deodorant. You don't need to give up makeup, nail polish, or moisturizers. There are products available that are nontoxic and better for your health. Once you know what you're looking for, you'll find a wide selection of aluminum-free deodorants, triclosan-free mouthwashes, fluoride-free toothpastes, and nontoxic sunscreens, moisturizers, shampoos, and other hair care products. The Resource Guide at the end of the book will help you find safe non- or less toxic replacements. I have even shared some of my favorite products.

> Check out the Environmental Working Group's website (www.ewg.org) and their awesome new app called SkinDeep. These two sources will allow you to search through all your lotions, creams, soaps, cleaners, and so on, discover which ones are toxic, and find safe brands.

How the Stark Naked 21-Day Metabolic Reset and Lifestyle Support Your Liver

The Stark Naked 21-Day Metabolic Reset uses a number of naturally proven ways to support your liver. First, we will be removing our three high-achieving lifestyle addictions—coffee, alcohol, and sugar. It is critical to remove these for the initial 21-day period, because they are each a major burden on your liver. Additional ways that are non-supplement-driven include drinking warm lemon water first thing in the morning to stimulate your liver, removing protein- and fat-based breakfasts that are hard on a sluggish liver, and extending the detoxification period by replacing a solid breakfast with a green smoothie that supports the liver. (I get into this in greater detail in Chapter 11.) You will also be reducing your fat intake for the initial 21 days, so your liver can catch up on metabolizing the stored, clogged fat. You have to do everything you can to give your liver a break while you are using the natural liver-aid solutions in the Reset period. If you don't, the Reset won't be as effective, and you will have wasted your precious time and energy only removing the new toxins entering your body and not clearing the ones stored in your fat.

If you drink a lot of coffee, you will notice two things early in the Reset. First, you're going to have a nasty headache for the first few days. Second, you are going to be crazy hungry. The headache is obvious and expected because of the caffeine withdrawal, but why the major increase in appetite? Is this a starvation diet?

The answer is no! This is not a deprivation diet. In fact, I'd prefer it if you didn't think of it as a diet at all.

You will be hungry because coffee is a major appetite suppressant. Without it, you are going to find yourself constantly thinking about food for the first few days. During my most recent reset with my wife, I was so unbelievable hungry and grumpy during the first 5 days; no matter how much protein and how many vegetables I ate, I couldn't be satisfied. I was constantly focused on my watch, counting down the seconds until I could eat my next meal.

But by day 7 everything changed. I was easily satisfied in between meals. Once the initial rough period was over, it became much easier to stay the course for the remainder of the 21 days. Yes, even I had to tolerate those first few days, but it was worth it. The rougher it is in the beginning, the better the results you usually see in the end.

To make it worth your while to suffer through those first rough days, focus on the benefits of cleaning up your liver. You will have more energy, the most valuable benefit of this program. Well, maybe the second most valuable. I've yet to have anyone complain about an increased sex drive! When your energy is up, your drive and hunger for life are elevated; everyone actually enjoys being around you and is inspired by you. Increased energy also means energy to have more sex. Exercise is actually enjoyable when you have more energy. Trust me, raw energy created from a revved-up, healthy metabolism blows caffeine-driven energy out of the water every time. There is no comparison—not even close!

Other benefits related to improved liver function are healthier, younger looking skin, better bowel movements, breath that doesn't smell as bad, early morning energy, fewer hot flashes, less body fat around the hips and thighs, a more stable mood, better brain clarity and focus, and improved sleep. Did I mention improved sex drive? Of course I did! What do you expect? I'm a guy, and we think about sex every 7 seconds.

Look, the bottom line is that if you want to get the most out of the Reset, you will commit to aggressively supporting your liver for the next 21 days. You will commit to no coffee, alcohol, or sugar without grumbling about it. In fact, maybe you'll even welcome the break. Just follow the Reset. If you do, the sky is the limit for your results, especially once your liver is back on your side of the field.

Love your liver during the 21-Day Reset by removing the three major toxins causing it to become sluggish and following the other liver-supporting elements of the Reset fundamentals in Chapter 11 (see page 204).

5. No coffee.

6. No alcohol.

7. Remove sugar from your diet—all sources of sugar.

4

Healthy Foods Gone Rogue

The Impact of Food Sensitivities and Food-Induced Inflammation

A FTER A HIGH-STRESS LIFESTYLE and liver toxicity, the final catalyst that triggers the Metabolic Breakdown Cycle is something most of you have likely never heard about, but it's probably the biggest reason you are not seeing the results you want with your current nutrition plan—*inflammation brought on by food sensitivities.*

Even if you believe you've been eating a healthy diet, you might be eating the wrong foods *for you,* foods that are causing inflammation and discomfort in the gut and other symptoms you're not connecting to what you're eating. By now you realize stress is negatively impacting your health, and you've likely heard about or have even tried the latest and greatest detoxification programs that promise to bring balance and harmony back to your liver. But how many of you have removed foods that you are sensitive to from your eating plan? Even if you're eating fruits, vegetables, and minimally processed foods, you might still be eating all of the wrong foods *for you,* and that could be causing your body stress.

Eliminating food sensitivities is a key component of the success of the Stark Naked 21-Day Metabolic Reset. Understanding the importance and role food sensitivities play in our digestion and health has single-handedly changed more lives than any other strategy we use at Stark. It is so powerful that I am shocked it hasn't become a more mainstream medical protocol.

Chris Speicher, cofounder of Speicher Group,
   a real-estate firm
Maryland
Age forty-three

▶ *Chris was introduced to the Reset when my client real-estate coach Tom Ferry challenged a number of his clients to try it. At first, Chris was leery, because he had major stomach and bowel issues. He couldn't sleep through the night without having to use the bathroom. He was always nervous about eating out in restaurants, because he didn't know what the bathroom situation would be like. He even hated going to concerts and sporting events for the very same reason. He had lived this way for over twenty years.*

No matter what he ate, he always felt sick afterward. He described the feeling as similar to constantly being nervous. He also suffered from severe and chronic joint pain.

Chris had tried everything to combat his condition over the years, following different diets, only eating vegetables, not eating vegetables, and so on, but nothing provided relief. He was constantly taking antacids and had recently finished a six-month dose of antibiotics prescribed by a gastrointestinal doctor. Still no relief. No doctor could figure out the cause of his discomfort, and no medication could seem to fix it. Chris believed he was going to live the rest of his life like this. He certainly didn't believe the Reset would help, but he had nothing to lose by trying it.

His response to the Reset was immediate and life-changing.

To figure out an individual's exact food sensitivities, an expensive lab test called the Mediator Release Test (MRT) is usually administered. The MRT is a blood test that looks at how your body responds to 150 different foods and chemicals and accounts for all reactions by noting the presence of chemical mediators, such as histamines, cytokines, and prostaglandins, released by your immune cells. A blind

Within the first couple of days, Chris felt a natural cleansing taking place. One week into the program his stomach issues had almost completely subsided. His joint pain went away, and his energy level skyrocketed.

By the end of week two, Chris had experienced his first week of solid bowel movements in more than two decades. He was committed to changing his eating habits for the rest of his life.

Why did he see these results?

Eating the wrong foods, even foods deemed healthy, was causing major inflammation and destroying his digestive tract. By simply removing those foods through the Reset, his symptoms began to quickly subside.

Being able to enjoying dinners out with his wife and sporting events with his buddies and not living in fear of the nearest bathroom gave Chris back his life. He has stuck to the approved-foods list in Phase 2, and his life is dramatically different than it used to be. He has not had any major digestive issues since starting the Reset. He feels healthier and more confident than ever. His clothes fit better, and he now sleeps like a rock—something he had struggled with his entire adult life.

At forty-three, Chris has taken up power lifting, and his strength over the last year has dramatically improved. His improved digestion is allowing him to rebuild muscle tissue and recover from his intense training, causing amazing results. Chris truly feels unstoppable!

peer-reviewed scientific study showed the MRT to have the highest level of accuracy of any food-sensitivity blood test (94.5 percent sensitivity and 91.8 percent specificity).

Thankfully, our clients are in pursuit of the ultimate energy and performance edge, so the majority of them have taken the MRT. When we get their lab results, we know exactly which foods to remove from their diet based on their sensitivity level.

I know what you're thinking. "Sure, you can have your clients take an expensive blood test. But I can't do that. I don't have the money, and my insurance won't pay for that!"

Guess what? You don't need to take the MRT. I've done the work for you!

So how can I remove the foods you are sensitive to without making you take the expensive blood test? Over the years, we have collected enough data to know the most common food sensitivities. I personally went through every one of our clients' MRTs from the last several years and tallied every food sensitivity. Based on that information, we've removed the foods from the Reset diet plan and compiled a list of approved foods for the 21-Day Reset period. Although this approach may not create an individualized list of food sensitivities for you, I guarantee most offending foods will be pulled from your diet on the Reset.

How can I be so confident?

The results speak for themselves. The approximately fifteen hundred people who have done the Reset and eaten only from the approved-foods list have seen tremendous results, including losing weight—anywhere between 8 and 20 pounds—feeling great, having

The Stark Naked 21-Day Metabolic Reset does not focus on removing immunoglobulin E (IgE) food allergens from the approved-foods list. If you know you have a food allergy, leave that food out of your diet.

more energy, sleeping better, experiencing less bloating and gas, and having greater mojo.

Removing foods you are sensitive to while reducing stress and supporting your liver leads to amazing results!

The Impact of Food Sensitivities on Your Body

First, it's important to understand that food sensitivities are not food allergies. They both cause inflammation, but food allergies are serious reactions that create what's called an immunoglobulin E (IgE) response from your immune system. When you ingest something that you are allergic to, such as peanuts, eggs, milk, or shellfish, your immune system releases what's called IgE antibodies to attack the allergen. This can produce symptoms in multiple areas of the body including your eyes (tearing, redness, itchiness), nose (discharge, itchiness, congestion), throat (tightness), lungs (shortness of breath, cough), skin (hives, swelling), or GI tract (vomiting, nausea) and trigger anaphylaxis, a severe whole-body allergic reaction. If untreated, anaphylaxis can kill you.

Food sensitivities also trigger your immune system, but not in a way that uses IgE. When you consume a food you're sensitive to, your immune cells are stimulated to release several different chemicals called chemical mediators. Some of the most well-known chemical mediators are histamine, cytokine, and prostaglandin. These cause a negative response in your body and symptoms such as migraine headaches, acid reflux, bloating, foggy thinking, depression, irritable bowel syndrome (IBS), asthma, arthritis, attention deficit disorder (ADD), and weight gain.

Unlike IgE food allergies, food sensitivities do not cause an immediate negative reaction in the body. Food-sensitivity symptoms can show up anywhere from 45 minutes to 3 days after you eat! With that kind of span in between meals, how in the world are you supposed to figure out the true culprit causing your symptoms? Was it what you ate for breakfast yesterday or what you had for lunch today that is causing you discomfort this evening?

Whenever I talk to people about food sensitivities for the first time, the classic response is usually, "I am completely fine with all types of food! There are no foods that bother me." I usually snicker whenever I hear that, because over time I have learned that most of us have grown so accustomed to feeling lousy that we are oblivious to the foods that are causing issues in our bodies.

The body is built in a special way to deal with small stressors that are constant, but not life-threatening. That is basically what these food sensitivities are: small stressors that affect the body, but are not considered life-threatening.

I spent the early years of my life growing up on a dairy farm in McMinnville, Oregon, and it was always funny to watch people's initial response when they got out of the car to visit us. The smell of manure overwhelmed their senses. It was all they could focus on initially, but the longer they hung around, the less the smell bothered them. That is, until they left the farm and then came back. Watching that initial reaction never got old.

Like those visitors, you've become used to your offenders and their negative impact on your body. They're just a normal part of your life. Before I took my first MRT, I experienced this firsthand—on the day I proposed to my wife. It was a perfect California day—blue skies and sunshine. My wife awoke to roses and loose rose petals all over our bed and bedroom floor, with a trail of flowers leading her out of the bedroom to where I was surrounded by bouquets of roses and coffee from her favorite coffee shop. I got down on bended knee and somehow successfully persuaded her to say yes!

We decided to have a nice relaxed lunch midday, and I ordered my favorite meat, beef. As usual, my left eye began to water. This happened often, which I was told was due to seasonal allergies. It was something I had become so used to that I didn't think much about it and made a mental note to pop an allergy pill when we got home.

I surprised my wife at lunch with our plans for the evening: dinner with our close friends at Club 33, a private restaurant in Disneyland. She was superexcited. We went home to get ready for our big night. My left eye was still watering like crazy when we arrived at Disneyland. I had forgotten to take an allergy pill! I was miserable!

When our friends arrived, they were 20 minutes late and cautiously asked us if everything was okay. I thought that was a weird question to ask a couple who just got engaged. During dinner they finally confessed that they were late because, as they were walking up to meet us, they noticed my left eye watering so badly they thought I was crying. They actually thought my wife had turned down my proposal! They literally walked around the park in circles for 20 minutes trying to decide what they should do!

After taking the MRT, I discovered beef was one of the foods I was sensitive to. By removing it from my diet and then reintroducing it, I've discovered that it is beef that makes my left eye water really badly—not seasonal allergies. For too long I thought I had watery eyes and my only recourse for relief was an allergy pill, when in fact my misery was actually being triggered by a food I was eating every day.

What are other symptoms that can be caused by food sensitivities?

Food sensitivities can affect you in multiple ways. They can create digestive complaints like bloating, diarrhea, constipation, IBS, GERD (acid reflux), and abdominal pain. They can cause fatigue and insomnia. They have been linked to depression, anxiety, irritability, and brain fog. They can cause food cravings and water retention, leading to weight gain, and metabolic syndrome, a cluster of symptoms that increase your risk of cardiovascular disease and type 2 diabetes. These symptoms include high blood pressure, high fasting glucose levels, excess fat gain around your belly, and elevated cholesterol levels. Food sensitivities have also been linked to problems with your skin, sinus and nasal issues, and joint pain. Reduced joint pain and enhanced brain function are two of the most common results people rave about after doing the Reset.

Now do you understand why addressing food sensitivities is such a necessary and essential component to your overall success?

How the Stark Naked Metabolic 21-Day Reset and Lifestyle Reduce Food-Induced Inflammation

The food we eat is used for a whole lot more than just energy. It forms the building blocks of your metabolism. It is used to rebuild tissue, make hormones, and replenish neurotransmitters in the brain. If your digestion is not working properly, you're going to have a hard time assimilating the foods you eat, and your metabolism will suffer the consequences.

A major disruptor of good digestion is food your body is sensitive to. These foods may be considered healthy food choices, but if your body sees them as a threat, it will trigger your immune system, cause systemic inflammation, and release the stress hormone cortisol.

Eating what you think of as healthy foods—fruits, vegetables, nuts, whole grains—may not be giving you the fuel you need to reach your peak performance. If you are sensitive to a "healthy" food, it's causing inflammation and damaging your body. When you see the approved-foods list for the Reset, you will most likely be surprised at the foods that do not appear on it. During the Reset you will avoid blueberries, shrimp, most nuts, broccoli, and salmon, for example. These are just some of the foods that routinely cause inflammation for my clients.

I'll wait while you go back and read that list again.

I have a friend who didn't want to take the MRT, because he was afraid the only two foods he actually eats salmon and almonds, would be on his list of sensitivities. "What will I eat?" he asked.

I need you to understand that I am not saying these foods are unhealthy. They're not, and that would be ridiculous. They're very healthy foods, packed with essential nutrients and vitamins, but for you they may be triggering inflammation and causing problems. By eliminating these foods for a period of time, you'll be able to tell if you are sensitive to them. You have got to get away from the foods you are sensitive to and give your body a break from these non-life-threatening stressors.

Here's the good news. The elimination period is only 21 days! In Phase 2 when I show you how to optimize your metabolism, I will teach you how to reintroduce foods you are jonesing to have back in your diet to see if they are safe or still a problem. You will know the answer right away. You see, when you remove a trigger food from your diet for a period of time and then reintroduce it, if it's still a problem, it will be like going back to the dairy farm. You will be amazed at how severe the symptoms are that you had originally become so numb to.

"How in the world did I end up with these sensitivities in the first place?" is a very common question people ask, once they experience the difference eliminating trigger foods can make in their life. There is still a lot left for us to learn about how these sensitivities develop, but three of the most common ways suggested by research are genetics, overexposure (eating the same thing over and over), and chronic stress. There is that word "stress" again!

By following the Reset, you will reduce unneeded chronic stress loads. This relieves the burden on your gut and creates an ideal environment for it to improve.

The role of genetics is an interesting one and something we have studied a lot at Stark. We use a few different genetic tests to help us construct high-performance plans for our clients after they have rebooted their health by resetting their metabolism. When it comes to genetics Dr. Mehmet Oz said it best: "Genes load the gun, lifestyle pulls the trigger." You are far from doomed by your genetics. It's your lifestyle that causes the majority of your problems. You choose how you live. Knowing there are some foods you will never be able to tolerate makes things a lot easier. Those foods will always be a trigger for you, regardless of how long you stay away from them.

Overexposure is a major contributor to food sensitivity. Why?

Most of us like routine. Do you have the same thing for breakfast every morning? Or, like the friend I mentioned earlier, only eat a few foods? In this case, there can be too much of a good thing. I believe this is the reason so many of my clients are sensitive to foods like blueberries, almonds, salmon, and broccoli. These are all known "power foods" for your health, so they went into overachiever mode and ate them—all the time. Instead of incorporating them into a balanced diet full of variety, they decided to eat these foods every single day to be superhealthy.

Brendan Steele, professional golfer
California
Age thirty-one

▶ Brendan Steele, a PGA Tour golfer, came to me at the end of his 2012 season, because he wanted to put some weight on to help increase his strength for driving distance and improve his durability to reduce back pain. Brendan was a slender 6 foot 2 and 172 pounds, but during our initial meeting and evaluation his body fat came out high for his size, and I noticed his lower stomach was very distended. I asked Brendan how his digestion was, and he responded that he had struggled with it for some time, but he had learned to just deal with it. I explained to Brendan that if he truly wanted to put on good muscle mass that is usable in his sport he had to get incredibly healthy first, and having bad digestion would prevent any possibility of that. Most people don't understand the importance of good digestion.

It's amazing how many people actually struggle to put weight on. The Stark Naked 21-Day Metabolic Reset is not just for weight loss. It can also help people just like Brendan who need to put on weight.

We ran the MRT on Brendan to determine his food sensitivities and discovered he was sensitive to most of what he was eating! We had to completely revamp Brendan's diet. We started by hav-

If you're a true creature of habit who eats the same food day in and day out, even healthy food, you may be doing more harm than good by eating the same foods over and over without giving your system a break. If this sounds like you, now you know why the perfect diet of superfoods may be making you feel so lousy. Your body was not built to function on the same foods every day. It was built for variety.

To receive these amazing benefits of removing foods you are sensitive to, you just have to simply follow the approved-foods list for 21

ing him eat only from the approved-foods list of the Reset. We had to give his body time to heal itself. Whether you need to lose weight or put weight on, you have to start by fixing what's broken! Brendan had to have faith in me, because I knew he would initially drop a lot of weight in the first 21 days, and that was far from his goal. But that was bad weight, and it was holding him back from making progress.

His body continued to heal itself in Phase 2, and during the initial few months his weight dropped all the way to 160 pounds. This was not the outcome Brendan was looking for, but he remained patient with me and his trust and patience have paid off incredibly. Eighteen months later he now weighs 190 pounds, and his body fat is very low. Brendan has lost 10 pounds of fat and added 30 pounds of muscle over two full PGA Tour seasons. His newfound muscle mass and strength has added 8 miles per hour to his club-head speed, and his average driving distance has improved by over 20 yards. That's incredible improvement for an athlete already playing at the highest level of a sport. He also has not missed one round of golf due to back pain in over two seasons. When we started working together two years ago he was ranked 205th, and for the first time in his ten-year professional career he broke into the top 100 world rankings. And he's still climbing. Not a bad jump!

days. Don't veer from it, don't ask to make any changes, just stick to it for 21 days. It's simple. If it's on the list, you can eat it. If it's not on the list, you can't eat it.

For example, beans and lentils are not on the list for the first 21 days, so please avoid them. I have found that beans are a major cause of inflammation in a lot of people. The main reason for this is that beans and lentils contain oligosaccharides. Oligosaccharides are a complex sugar that is very challenging for humans to digest. Many experts believe the reason is that we either don't make the enzyme alpha-galactosidase needed to break oligosaccharides down or only make very small amounts. When oligosaccharides are present in the gut and the enzyme needed to break them down is either absent or in short supply, you end up with bloating, cramping, and unwanted gas.

That experience may be fun for kids ("Beans, beans, the musical fruit, the more you eat, the more you toot"), but for most adults it usually leads to embarrassment. Another reason to avoid beans is because they contain phytic acid, which can strip our body of essential minerals. Truth be told, we don't need any extra help chasing away more minerals. My goal is to help you retain the good stuff! So, for the Reset, stay away from the beans.

Last, if there is a food you know you have issues with and it's on the list of approved foods, please don't force yourself to eat it. Go ahead and keep it out of your diet.

Even if you believe you've been eating a healthy diet, you might be eating the wrong foods for you, which are causing inflammation and discomfort in the gut and other symptoms. During the Reset, you'll avoid the foods shown to cause the most inflammation and use other lifestyle strategies to get the most from your food (see page 204).

8. Follow the list of approved foods.

5

Warning! Danger Ahead

Why You Have Low Mojo

OH, YEAH, I'M GOING THERE. I am treading into territory few are willing to explore, and yet so many of you are dealing with it. I'm talking about not having sex. As a personal trainer, I hear all sorts of intimate details about my clients' lives, but the topic that seems to creep up more often than expected is a question many deal with and so few admit: "What in the world has happened to my mojo?"

You may be wondering why I find this an important topic to talk about in a book about health and fitness. I mean, isn't lack of sexual desire just part of getting older? *No!*

If you remember back to the Metabolic Breakdown Cycle, chronic stress leads to altered hormones, eventually leading to a lethargic metabolism. If your sex drive has disappeared, that's a huge warning sign that you are in the midst of a metabolic breakdown and on your way to hitting rock bottom. You may not have had a total breakdown yet, but believe me, untreated, you are well on your way.

If your mojo is not what it used to be, you are going to need to commit to the Stark Naked 21-Day Metabolic Reset, and fast, or you will suffer the consequences of a total breakdown, making it much harder for you to reset later. The Reset alone won't be enough to recharge worn-out sex hormones. It's going to take a full lifestyle overhaul and lots of catching up on lost sleep, so make sure to pay attention to Chapter 8, the sleep chapter, because sleep will become your greatest ally. But believe me, if it means getting your groove back, it's worth it.

When it comes to lost or low mojo, I find that most men either overcompensate by excessively bragging about their sexuality to their friends or clam up and say nothing at all, because in their mind their lack of sex drive equals a loss in manhood.

On the other hand, I find women openly discuss their loss of interest in sex or lack of attraction to their mate, as if it is a rite of passage with age. Most women past the age of thirty-five who are clients at Stark will readily admit that they know something is wrong with their hormones. They inherently understand something is off kilter and their sex drive is different than it once was. It's amazing how many women I see in the gym who say they'd rather knit than have sex with their spouse.

Has it really gotten that bad that you would rather knit than engage in the horizontal tango? Trust me! Life is better when sex is at the center of it.

Here's something to think about. If you would rather sleep than have sex, consider yourself closer to death than life.

In the movie *40 Days and 40 Nights* a young twenty-something played by Josh Hartnett vows to go 40 days and 40 nights without having sex to make himself a better man, a decision that almost kills him. When I was younger, 40 days of no sex felt like an eternity, but when I was beat down to a lethargic pulp, 40 days was an easy conquest. Did it make me a better man? Far from it—just ask my wife!

I was miserable and unmotivated in every area of life. Sex was the last thing on my mind when my total testosterone levels came in at 102 nanograms per deciliter (ng/dL)—a third of the normal low (300 ng/dL). These days, at forty, can I go sexless 40 days without dying? Yes, but it's far from ideal or my idea of a good time!

My wife recently had our third child, and her pregnancy was a challenging one. When she first announced that she was pregnant, I was excited, because that usually means an increased sex drive, but that dream was short-lived. This pregnancy, she was sicker than sick nearly every day for the first twenty weeks. There wasn't much hanky-panky between us during that period—and, of course, I understood. Naturally, I found a way to survive. You can bet that when the few opportunities did appear, I definitely rose to the occasion! Though, looking back, I honestly think my wife was taking pity on me. Us men—we really are such babies!

My wife figured me out very early in our relationship. If she wanted me to move mountains, she was very strategic in how she motivated me. When it came to our sex life, she realized I couldn't get enough of her; nine years later I still can't! It's one of the great perks of marriage that comes with healthy hormones. My wife knows exactly how to use her charm to motivate me to do anything—even hang the Christmas lights. She doesn't have to nag me! Nope. All she needs to do is come home with some mistletoe, put it over my head, give me an intense kiss and her sexy, seductive look, and I am putty. Those bad boys are usually hung in an hour!

Now, if you're a married man like me, we all know our women have the ability to get us with their womanly ways, but the truth is, anyone in a relationship understands that bringing home flowers for no reason, planning a surprise weekend away from the kids, cooking a romantic dinner for two, cleaning the house, or just about any small unexpected gesture goes a really long way with our significant other. I know my wife loves it when I give her time away from the kids, a night out with her girlfriends, a massage in bed that *isn't* meant to be foreplay (okay, maybe it is), or a foot rub after a long run or hike we took together. Sure, I know these things usually lead to the horizontal mambo, but I also know they make my wife happy. And as the saying goes, "Happy wife, happy life!"

But what happens when the fire goes out? When, no matter how hard you stoke the flames, there is no fire? What the hell happened? Where has your desire for sex gone?

Most of us believe a shrinking sex drive comes with aging, but I don't buy that and I don't like when I hear clients use that as an excuse. I train a couple in their mid-seventies who have sex at least two or three times a week. During a workout, the wife once inquired whether I knew of any supplements to slow her husband down a bit. "He wants it all the time!" she said.

She went on to explain that if he simply sees a small flash of any of her bare skin, he's all over her and won't stop until she gives in and has sex with him. I can tell she loves that he still pursues her so passionately at seventy-five years of age and he doesn't need Viagra to make it happen.

Guess what? That's the potential we *all* have when we take proper care of ourselves!

I believe we are supposed to still be enjoying sex late in life. Now that I am in my forties, I am convinced that I am just reaching my sexual prime, despite research to the contrary that says men reach their sexual prime much younger. When I was thirty-three, I wouldn't have believed that was possible. I had just come off training with the U.S. bobsled team, so my body looked amazing. According to my wife, I had the physique of a Greek god. I was 5 foot 10, I weighed 205 pounds, and my body fat was under 10 percent. When I looked like that, one would have assumed I had a sex drive that was through the roof. But I didn't. In fact, my mojo was so low that I would rather have slept than had sex. My greatest desire in life was sleep. This was not healthy for a man my age or for my marriage.

We are always told not to judge a book by its cover, and I was a walking, talking example of that back then. Just because the outside looked good, it didn't mean the insides were functioning as they should. I have seen more perfectly chiseled high achievers with destroyed hormones than those with optimal hormones. Sadly, it is usually the best-looking men and women who I find have done the most damage to themselves. Remember, fitness can mask health.

We live in a world where we are constantly told that if we exercise (a lot), eat superclean, and get really lean, we are guaranteed to have optimal hormone levels. With the optimal hormone levels, we are guaranteed to desire more sex. Right?

Wrong!

In his groundbreaking book *Why Zebras Don't Get Ulcers,* Robert Sapolsky discusses in detail how stress negatively affects sex hormones in men and women. In fact, it's such an important topic, he writes an entire chapter on it. I am going to give you a basic understanding of how stress (have you noticed a pattern here yet?) is the main culprit that is likely shutting down your sex drive. If you don't deal with reducing your stress load—and I mean now—your hormones will never operate at an optimal level.

How Stress Robs Men of Their Desire for Sex

When it comes to men and sex, our hormones, just like our needs in life, are really very simple. Testosterone is a great predictor of biological aging in men. When testosterone dips, we suffer—a lot. This decrease can affect everything from our sexual desires to the ability to get it up, our general state of happiness, our drive in life, and our body fat, muscle mass, and mental concentration; it can dramatically increase the risk of an early death.

Basically the higher your testosterone level, the younger you are on the inside. Conversely, the lower it is, the older you are, independent of your actual age. The *Journal of Clinical Endocrinology and Metabolism* published a study following 794 men from the San Diego area over the age of fifty. It found that at an 11.8-year follow-up the men with the lowest testosterone levels (less than 241 ng/dL) were 40 percent more likely to die than those with higher levels. Similarly, in an August 2006 article in the *Archives of Internal Medicine,* a team of

U.S. doctors determined that men over the age of forty had an 88 percent increased risk of death associated with low levels of testosterone. An *ABC News* article highlighted research from the New England Research Institute stating that one in four men over the age of thirty suffers from low testosterone. (I was one of them.)

The reference range for normal total testosterone is usually 300–1000 ng/dL; anyone with levels under 300 ng/dL is considered to have low testosterone. This is a huge range in my opinion. I can personally testify that at 1000 ng/dL sex is all you can think about, but at 300 ng/dL Megan Fox hardly catches your attention. What's frightening in this research is the direction most men's testosterone levels are headed in general. By the year 2025, researchers are predicting a 38 percent increase in men between the ages of thirty and seventy-nine who are plagued with low testosterone. Something has to change, or it won't be long before a majority of men are suffering from low testosterone and being robbed of their best possible lives. The scariest part for most men is that one of the last things to go in their health decline is their sex drive and the ability to get it up. By the time they reach that point, they're pretty jacked up. I believe that's why there is an elevated risk of early death associated with low testosterone in older men.

Why is this happening?

Your brain is the control center for producing the majority of your hormones. In Chapter 2 we explored its role in triggering the stress hormones that unleash your inner Hulk and keep you alive in times of trouble. It is also responsible for producing more sex hormones. With a healthy metabolism, when your brain receives signals that your mojo is running low, it sends signals to your testes to produce more testosterone and refill your mojo. It is programmed to keep your sex hormones in a balanced state at all times, so you function at an optimal level and desire sex.

The major issue impacting your mojo in this day and age is likely chronic stress. So what happens when your body is under stress?

As soon as the brain perceives stress and signals the release of your stress hormones, the whole system for making sex hormones is shut down. Consequently there is an immediate reduction in mojo-making hormones. The production process for these sex hormones cannot be flipped back on until the stress-response system is calmed down. A 2011 study conducted by the University of California, Berkeley, supports the correlation between stress and the shutdown of the sex drive.

When you think about it, it makes perfect sense. The desire to reproduce is the second most important of the human drives.

Do you recall the first?

To survive at all costs!

A beautiful woman can make men do all sorts of crazy things, and our bodies know it, so to keep the focus on survival in the face of danger, the reproductive drives are shut down.

So, let's say it's the year 2040, and you're facing a zombie apocalypse. Out of self-preservation, you've suddenly found yourself in a fight-or-flight mode because you are running from a zombie. Your body will automatically shut down the desire for sex to protect you. I don't care if Elle MacPherson or Brooklyn Decker crosses your path—when you are running for your life, you are not going to stop and ask the zombie for a time-out to try and score. Believe it or not, you won't even want to.

It has also been discovered that it's not just life-or-death stressors that cause this reduction-in-testosterone response. It's all kinds of daily stressors, including pain, illness, poor eating habits, psychological stress, emotional stress, lack of sleep, excessive alcohol, and even overexercising, that can easily slow down your testosterone production. Yes, you read that right—too much exercise bashes and beats your mojo into submission.

Take it from a guy who knows firsthand. That's what happened to me in my early thirties. I had overtrained and, without realizing it, overstressed myself into a state where I had severely low testosterone levels. Now let me follow up by saying that I know exercise in the right proportion is a great thing. But like everything in life, too much of a good thing—even exercise—can be damaging. Research is very clear that moderate exercise is great for our bodies, but extreme intense exercise can cause more harm than good. Experts have shown that when you combine a poor diet, lack of rest, and too much exercise, you drive that pesky stress hormone cortisol through the roof.

What is suppressed when cortisol is elevated? You guessed it! Your mojo.

For years I have said, "The more insane your exercise program, the more insane your nutrition and recovery strategies better be, or you're going to find yourself on the road to metabolic disaster." I don't want to see you headed on that path. I will give you great strategies for tracking and managing safe exercise and recovery in Chapter 9.

And if I haven't already made it clear, I am about to put the final nail in the coffin for you on how stress impacts your sex life. When you have low mojo, not only don't you feel like having sex, even if you do, your stress-signaling system is likely having a negative impact on your erections. In 2012 the drugs targeting erectile dysfunction were valued at $4.3 billion for the year. That's a lot of ED drugs driving erections.

So how is stress affecting your ability to get it up?

We know it takes an increase of blood flow to rise to your calling. A reduction in cardiovascular health is the major contributor to our limp-noodle epidemic, but stress can also prevent you from responding to your sexual calling. You have to be in a calm state to obtain and sustain an erection. If stress is elevated, it is difficult to get it up, and if by some chance you are able to, that stress response will most likely cause premature ejaculation. Every man has experienced premature ejaculation. Yeah, we joke about it, but most of us are hiding the truth that we have experienced the inability to either get it up prior to sex or keep it up, often because of nervousness during sex. That reality often deeply scars us with embarrassment and hang-ups that get into our heads, making it tougher to stay calm the next time a sexual encounter occurs.

Now that I've delivered the reasons for your low mojo, allow me to give you some good news. The Stark Naked 21-Day Metabolic Reset will dramatically improve your erections by drastically increasing your cardiovascular health and overall blood flow! (You can thank all of the green vegetables and water you'll be consuming for that!) It will also drastically reduce your overall stress load, making it much easier for you to relax before and during sex.

I bet when you bought this book, you weren't expecting this added bonus!

How Stress Robs Women of Sexual Desire

Buckle your seat belts, ladies. You're not immune either. We are going on the ultimate roller-coaster ride. Yes, we are going to talk about women's hormones, which are far more complicated than men's. They drastically change each month according to a woman's cycle. To make it even more confusing, birth control and menopause have dramatic effects on your hormones—and they're different for every woman. I could write an entire book on this subject, but for our purposes I am going to focus solely on estrogen, progesterone, and testosterone and the impact these three hormones have on a woman's body when they are out of balance. It can result in unnecessary fat gain, inexplicable depression, and even low sexual desire.

Understanding Estrogen and Progesterone

Ladies, stay with me here. This is a little more intense, but unlike us thick-headed, zero-attention-span men, I know you have the ability to absorb information at a deeper level, so I am going to dive in here with the hope that you want the information I am providing. I have met so many confused women over the years who feel miserable. They know their hormones are to blame, but are clueless about what's actually going on to create the way they feel.

In 2012 I had the opportunity to record a podcast with Robb Wolf, the author of *The Paleo Solution*, about how I help women balance their sex hormones to assist with fat loss. During my preparation for that interview, I came across an article by Dr. Jade Teta entitled "Female Phase Training: Training with the Female Cycle." The article discussed how to use different types of exercise in the different phases of a woman's cycle each month to create consistent fat loss. Dr. Teta's knowledge of women's sex hormones runs deep. As a result of reading that article, I reached out to him and have since developed a great personal friendship. Through my numerous conversations with Dr. Teta, I came to a better understanding of what women struggle with when dealing with unbalanced sex hormones and developed this Reset plan to help meet their needs.

Let's take a look at how your sex hormones are supposed to work and where the bulk of the chaos is coming from for most women.

Like a man's, your brain is also at the root of controlling and balancing your mojo hormones. However, in women the brain triggers different hormones at different times of the month. During the first half of your cycle the brain triggers the ovaries to produce estrogen; then it switches to triggering progesterone in the second half of your cycle. Your brain is also responsible for stimulating the ovaries to release eggs. Estrogen and progesterone perform a specific dance each month during your cycle, and they need to be in balance to work at their best.

During the follicular phase (days 1–14) of the cycle, estrogen is steadily rising while progesterone stays low. Estrogen peaks during ovulation, releasing a mature egg. Then during the luteal phase (days 15–28) the body increases production of progesterone, preparing the uterine wall for implantation of a fertilized egg. If fertilization of the egg does not happen, then both estrogen and progesterone dip at menses, and the process starts all over. When the cycle runs smoothly and the two hormones stay in balance, you breeze through your cycle sometimes surprised when your period shows up. You feel sexy and happy, you enjoy sex, PMS symptoms are almost nonexistent, and your waistline stays nice and trim. You and your significant other get the most out of life enjoying your sexy hourglass figure.

Estrogen Dominance

How many of you truly experience a regular monthly cycle?

Here's a fun idea. Ask your significant other what it's honestly like dealing with you during "that time of the month." Does your significant other strategically plan business trips around those few days every month? That could be a good sign your hormones are a bit off.

Estrogen dominance is usually the main factor disrupting a healthy monthly cycle. Estrogen dominance occurs when progesterone is deficient compared to estrogen. Some experts believe it's likely that as much as 50 percent of all menstruating women deal with estrogen dominance. That means one out of every two of you is dealing with hormones that are internally wreaking havoc, which can lead to symptoms like these from estrogen dominance:

- Anxiety
- Breast tenderness
- Bloating
- Depressed sex drive
- Fat gain around hips and thighs
- Fatigue
- Poor memory and foggy thinking
- Headaches
- Heavy bleeding during menstruation
- Irritability
- Insomnia

- Mood swings
- Enhanced PMS symptoms

If you experience some or all of these symptoms every month, there is a good chance you're dealing with estrogen dominance. If that's the case, it's time to take action.

When your hormonal balance is off so that estrogen is elevated and progesterone is too low, you will typically store excess fat on the hips and thighs and have a smaller waistline. This is due to estrogen's ability to prevent cortisol from storing weight gain around the waist, but experiencing estrogen dominance long enough will eventually lead to an expanding waistline as well. Most women notice this transitioning into menopause, as estrogen begins to decrease, leading to lower levels of both estrogen and progesterone and the resulting inability to offset cortisol and block fat accumulation around your midsection.

The first step to solving this problem is realizing that, just like for men, stress is at the root of the problem and the worst thing you can do is add more stress to the mix by attempting to eat less and exercise more. Your body has the ability to convert progesterone to cortisol to keep you alive, because survival is vital. Stress eventually causes progesterone to decrease, leading to estrogen dominance. Choosing to deprive yourself of food and punish your body with exercise as your weight-loss game plan creates too much of a stress response in your body, driving progesterone even farther downward and creating more estrogen dominance.

Over the years, I have met with many women whose hips and thighs have actually gotten bigger while their waistline has shrunk when they were eating less and exercising more, leaving them frustrated and angry. If that's how you are currently trying to overcome this problem, please do your body and sex drive a favor and stop!

You can't force the change! You have to fix the problem. You must first discover the cause of the imbalance.

There are three main culprits leading to estrogen dominance. Men, make sure you pay attention to this list, because it affects you too; estrogen dominance is becoming very common in men as well. Pay especially close attention to numbers 2 and 3 below. Estrogen buildup in men can lead to moobs (there it is again, that word for man boobs), fat gain around the hips and thighs, hair loss, loss of sex drive, impotence, hot flashes, and mood issues like irritability. There's a joke among my colleagues: it's not young, high-testosterone men who start wars; it's the crotchety, older estrogen-dominant men who trigger the wars and then send in their young testosterone-driven armies to finish what they started.

Source 1: The "Progesterone Steal" from Stress

Progesterone is considered by many to be the "mother of all hormones," because every other hormone in your body is made from it. When stress is elevated, the body can turn on what is known as "progesterone steal." When the adrenals are no longer able to keep up with the demand for cortisol production, the body has a backup plan to keep you going. That plan is to steal progesterone to keep your cortisol production moving.

Dr. Tina Marcantel explains this well in her article "Hormones and How They Interact": "Mother Progesterone feeds the loudest baby (cortisol), and the other children (DHEA [dehydroepiandrosterone, a natural steroid hormone], testosterone, and estradiol [an estrogen]) decrease in size because all the attention is being given to cortisol." Basically if your body is under stress and your brain is triggering the need for cortisol, your other hormones are going to suffer until the stress trigger is dampened. This is especially prevalent during states of adrenal burnout.

It's very common to find estrogen dominance issues in women who are exhausted from chronic stress exposure. This is also commonly seen during menopause and is one of the reasons a woman's waistline expands during menopause, even though her diet hasn't changed. Cortisol is stealing all the precursor building blocks of the sex hormones to keep it alive, and the other hormones (estrogen, progesterone, and testosterone) necessary to keep you skinny have been deprived so long, they barely exist anymore. Cortisol can be such a killjoy!

I have seen multiple women in their early forties showing signs of early menopause, and the one thing in common among all of them is their trashed adrenals from an overly stressed lifestyle.

Source 2: A Sluggish Liver

Another major player causing estrogen dominance is a sluggish liver. The liver is responsible for preventing estrogen from building up in your body. Estrogens are processed through the liver and shuttled out like all of the other toxins described in Chapter 3. When the liver is overwhelmed, the process of removing estrogens is slowed down, which causes estrogen to become stuck in the body. The result is that the estrogen side of the estrogen-to-progesterone ratio is elevated, leading to estrogen dominance, which causes you to experience the symptoms like fat storage on your hips and thighs, increased irritability, insomnia, fatigue, headaches, and foggy thinking.

To make matters even worse, when you combine low progesterone from stress with estrogen buildup due to a sluggish liver, you get that pesky Dr. Jekyll–Mr. Hyde monthly cycle. This is very common.

Now get this. The first line of defense for this hormonal imbalance recommended by our medical community is to add synthetic hormones to the mix in the form of a birth control pill, which is actually classified as a known carcinogen right along with tobacco and asbestos by the World Health Organization. Currently over eleven million U.S. women between the ages of fifteen and forty-four take oral birth control pills. Fifty-eight percent of users rely on the pill for other purposes besides pregnancy prevention. Some of the major reasons for use according to a 2011 Guttmacher Institute study: 31 percent use it for cramps or menstrual pain, 28 percent for menstrual regulation,

14 percent for acne. These are all symptoms of estrogen dominance.

I recently met with a young female athlete who was complaining of symptoms of estrogen dominance; specifically, she had a dramatic increase in body fat, and her PMS symptoms were noticeably rougher every month. After digging deeper into her medical history, I discovered she had symptoms of an extremely burdened liver. Four months prior to our first meeting she had stopped taking her birth control pills, because she felt they were making her too aggressive.

Unlike most women who are taking estrogen-based birth control pills, she was using the new form of birth control called Drospirenone (DRSP), which only contains progesterone. Remember, progesterone has the ability to convert into other hormones like cortisol. However, it can also convert to anabolic hormones like DHEA and testosterone. Although her birth control was doing a good job keeping her estrogen-progesterone balance in check, it was also allowing the excess progesterone to convert to anabolic hormones, making her significantly more aggressive. When she removed the birth control from her daily routine, her progesterone collapsed. Her elevated estrogen and a sluggish liver caused an extremely estrogen-dominant state. As a result, her body fat quickly elevated, especially around her hips and thighs. Her muscle mass and strength also diminished, and she went from being superaggressive to experiencing bouts of extreme anxiety, insomnia, and fatigue.

The Stark Naked 21-Day Metabolic Reset did wonders for her overwhelmed liver, allowing my client to drop 15 pounds in the first 21 days. For the first time in months, she was able to sleep again and no longer had mood swings or severe anxiety. She was able to fit back into her skinny clothes and had no severe PMS symptoms every month.

Source 3: Xenoestrogens (Environmental Estrogens)

In Chapter 3 we covered the chemicals you are exposed to from rubbing various beauty products onto your skin every day and the impact this has on your liver and sex hormones. One classification I want you to be aware of is xenoestrogens, synthetic chemicals that, once inside the body, can mimic estrogen. *Xeno,* from the Greek, means "foreign." We discussed parabens as an estrogen mimicker in Chapter 3, but there are additional environmental estrogens you are likely being exposed to. Other known xenoestrogens include:

Phthalates, commonly used in flooring and plastics and also found in perfumes, lotions, cosmetics, varnishes, nail polish.

Bisphenol A, found in the linings of most food and beverage cans and currently one of the highest-volume chemicals produced world- wide. The FDA has recently banned its use in baby bottles and infant formula.

Atrazine, an herbicide to control weeds, the second largest selling pesticide in the United States, banned in Europe in 2005. It is used on crops like corn and sugarcane and on golf courses and lawns.

Zeranol, currently used extensively as a growth stimulator in the beef and pork industries in the United States and Canada, banned in Europe in 1985.

Xenoestrogens are scary, and they are everywhere! Unless you want to remove yourself from society and go live deep in the wilder- ness of the Rockies, you are not going to escape xenoestrogens. The bottom line is this: you have to take the best measures to offset the damage these can cause. The Stark Naked 21-Day Metabolic Reset provides you with a good foundation of daily support to fight these substances, but you may wish to take your defense to another level and remove as many xenoestrogens from your lifestyle as possible.

Women and Testosterone

The last hormone I want to explore with you is testosterone, that scary manly hormone. Most women view testosterone as the hormone that creates gross-looking bulging muscles and hair in all the wrong places. Most of you want nothing to do with that bulky look. Trust me, I am not a fan either. More recently the role of elevated testosterone in polycystic ovary syndrome (PCOS) is another reason you want nothing to do with testosterone. Yes, testosterone is the primary hormone for men, and yes, high testosterone is associated with PCOS, but when testosterone drops in women it wreaks havoc within your body. It plays a major role in sexuality, helping with sexual desire and preparing you for sex with natural responses such as vaginal lubrication. When testosterone is too low, you no longer want sex, and if you have it, it's not especially enjoyable.

Low testosterone in women has been associated with the following symptoms:

- Anxiety
- Loss of libido
- Lethargy and lack of motivation
- Loss of muscle and strength
- Inability to climax
- Depression and mood swings
- Increased fat around your belly
- Elevated risk of osteoporosis
- Hair loss on the head and body

What causes low testosterone in women? The majority of testosterone for women is created by the adrenals. And though I realize I am starting to sound like a broken record, it cannot be overstated that the biggest culprit causing low testosterone in women is stress. When your adrenals have been mobilized to defend against stress, they are not allowed to replenish testosterone until the stress goes away.

Another very common trigger for low or reduced testosterone is the birth control pill. The pill works so well, it not only prevents you from getting pregnant; it actually reduces your desire to have sex in the first place by blunting testosterone. Last but not least, menopause is also another common cause of low testosterone. When a woman hits menopause, all hormones come crashing down, especially testosterone.

It's absurd how your current lifestyle is destroying your hormones, isn't it?

I hope testosterone just got a little less scary for you. If you're experiencing some of the symptoms talked about in this chapter, please follow the Stark Naked 21-Day Metabolic Reset exactly as it is laid out. It will be the start your body needs to revitalize your testosterone, rebalance your estrogen and progesterone levels, and give you back your swagger. If you choose to ignore these warning signs or, worse, if you have pushed yourself too hard for so long that not only are you dealing with a lot of these symptoms, but you are also exhausted all the time, you have entered the final stage of the Metabolic Breakdown Cycle, known as adrenal burnout.

> If your sex drive has disappeared, that's a huge warning sign that you are in the midst of a metabolic breakdown and on your way to hitting rock bottom. The Reset will help you get your mojo back.

6

The Consequences of
Your Metabolic Breakdown

The Dangers of Adrenal Burnout
and Hitting Rock Bottom

DO YOU WAKE UP FEELING TIRED? I mean inexplicably tired—as though you haven't slept enough, or at all, and you fear you can't make it through your day, even when you had 8 hours of sleep the night before? Or at the end of the day, are you so exhausted you can't make it through to the end of a movie without falling asleep?

Are you so tired that you are lacking your once virile sex drive? Do you suddenly experience random sugar or salt cravings you've never had before, feel depressed, or get sick all of the time? Do you find yourself uncontrollably irritable, unable to focus or remember things and basically lacking the joy and drive you once had in life?

If you answered yes to most (if not all) of these, you're in the final stage of the Metabolic Breakdown Cycle. You've definitely pushed too hard, too long, and your body has officially given up.

Welcome to the wonderful world of what is commonly referred to as adrenal burnout—meaning your adrenal glands are overworked and are functioning in a fatigued state. When the adrenals can no longer keep up, your body has basically given up its fight to keep you alive and has begun to shut down. Adrenal burnout has been a major buzzword in the world of high-performance athletes, but in the last few years it has become more mainstream among high achievers like you.

Most commonly associated with intense or prolonged stress, adrenal burnout occurs when the adrenal glands function below the necessary level. Your adrenal glands mobilize your body's responses to every kind of stress (whether it's physical, emotional, or psychological) through hormones that regulate energy production and storage, immune function, heart rate, muscle tone, and other processes. When your adrenals get fatigued, you have basically pushed yourself so hard for so long that the control system of the adrenals begins to wear out and shut down. Once they can't keep up with demands placed on them, you begin to suffer big-time.

Just about everything you do can and does impact your adrenals. If not managed properly and given enough rest, your adrenals will be overworked and forced to give up.

How do you know if you have hit the wall and are experiencing adrenal burnout?

Simple! Do you have any of these symptoms?

Getting light-headed when going from a lying to a standing position

Feeling overwhelmed

Hypoglycemia (low blood sugar)

Constant tiredness

Irritability and depression

Low blood pressure

Anxiety

Trouble staying asleep

Trouble getting out of bed in the morning

Lack of joy in life, everything is a struggle

Preference for sleep over sex

Severe brain fog and lack mental focus

No desire to exercise

If you are regularly experiencing three or more of these symptoms, then your adrenals are more than likely working in a state of adrenal burnout and your metabolism is seriously broken. Not only is the Stark Naked 21-Day Metabolic Reset an absolute must for you; your energy bank account is so far overdrawn, the bank is about to close your account unless you start replenishing the energy and fast!

I know this is going to be a tough adjustment for many of you, but the only exercise I recommend you do during the Stark Naked 21-Day Metabolic Reset is passive, such as taking walks in nature for 20 to 30 minutes a day. This is a secret recovery strategy I've learned the Russians use with their athletes. It's so secret they wouldn't even allow Ivan Drago to be shown doing it in *Rocky IV*. Okay, just kidding. It's not *that* secret, but you would be amazed who uses this strategy of walking in nature to enhance recovery and keep the metabolism running on all cylinders. Professional athletes, top CrossFit athletes, CEOs of very successful companies, U.S. Military Special Forces members, and yours truly take advantage of this strategy regularly. I will teach you how to use it to your advantage in Chapter 9, where I'll talk in greater detail about exercise during your reset.

In early January 2014, I received a phone call from the incredible world-class CrossFit athlete Becca Voigt. At age thirty-four, she has qualified for the brutally intense CrossFit Games seven years in a row and is recognized as one of the fittest women in the world. The CrossFit Games pride themselves on being the world's premier test of fitness. In 2014 over 140,000 people signed up for the CrossFit Open, hoping to earn a spot in the CrossFit Games. The 140,000 are eventually whittled down to the top 100 men and women in the world, who compete in multiple events challenging fitness and athleticism over a long weekend at the Home Depot Center in Los Angeles for the title "Fittest on Earth."

During our first conversation Becca told me she was suffering from adrenal burnout. She literally could not get out of bed in the mornings from excessive fatigue. She was emotionally worn out, lacking her usual drive for training and in life. Her necessary competition workouts were stalled, and her cardiovascular conditioning seemed to be slowly disappearing. Becca's body fat was suddenly elevated, and her old nutritional strategies of eating low-carb and superclean were no longer helping her usual six-pack or energy production. This was not a good sign. She asked me for my help to reset her system, so she could compete in the 2014 CrossFit Open that started in six weeks.

Things had to change for Becca, and they had to change fast! I quickly agreed with Becca's assessment that the biggest hurdle holding her back were her adrenals. They were definitely overworked and functioning in a burnout state. As with most overachieving athletes, I also found her liver very sluggish too. This combination can have a terrible impact on a high-performing athlete like Becca.

Our initial focus was to support her liver with strategies from the Reset while slowly increasing her carbohydrate intake to support her intense training volume, improving her body's ability to recover. How effective were these strategies?

Within two months, Becca went from struggling to get out of bed in the mornings to finishing second at the 2014 CrossFit Southern California Regionals and reaching her seventh straight CrossFit Games. If these strategies can rejuvenate someone like her, at the highest level of fitness competition, they can help any individuals reset their metabolism and get their adrenals back online—including *you*!

First, let's explore how you got here in the first place.

The Causes of Adrenal Burnout

Imagine for a moment that you are a race-car driver in the Indy 500. You're in total control of the car. You decide when to turn the steering wheel, apply the gas and brake, signal your pit crew that the car needs attention, and make pit stops for them to refuel and perform mechanical repairs. When your car is well cared for and finely tuned, the signal and demand system works smoothly, keeping your car operating at its peak performance and giving you your best chance of winning the big race.

Are you with me so far? In this analogy the driver is the brain, specifically the hypothalamus-pituitary complex (HP complex), the major control center for the glands that make hormones in your body. The hypothalamus connects your nervous system to your endocrine system through the pituitary gland and acts like a thermostat for your hormones. The hypothalamus receives input from your nervous system and triggers the pituitary to send specific signals to the different glands for hormone production and adjustments to keep them in balance, just like your thermostat regulates the temperature of your house.

A simple example of this is when the brain receives the input that you're moving from a lying to a standing position. The brain signals the adrenals to release epinephrine (adrenaline) to raise your blood pressure a little as you become erect. This happens in order to fight gravity and make sure blood stays in your brain, so you don't pass out. If your adrenals are exhausted and not working at optimum levels, you will feel light-headed and dizzy doing something as simple as going from lying to standing.

Think about that. Has this ever happened to you? If so, it might have been your body telling you your adrenals are running low on fuel just like a race car.

When your body, like the race car, is well cared for and finely tuned, it works at an optimum level, constantly maintaining a perfect balance to meet the performance demands. As the driver, you are constantly monitoring feedback from your car, correcting the positioning with your steering, applying the gas and the brakes at the right times to keep your car in the race around turns, and listening to your pit crew through radio communications. You're constantly getting feedback to keep you at your best.

But what happens when you decide to start ignoring feedback from the experts, thinking you know best? Trouble is waiting for you.

Let's say your tires signal you that it's time to make a pit stop and have them changed. Eager to stay in the race, you decide to override the signal. You decide that a pit stop isn't worth the time, so you fly right by the pit. Now things begin to get tough. The car is harder to control in the turns, but you know you can dig deep and overcome this with your superb driving skills. Next, you notice a warning light on your dash. It's the fuel gauge indicating that you'll need gas soon. Now, the smart thing to do would be to make a quick pit stop to change the tires and refuel, but no, you again override these signals, yet continue to demand that your car keep performing at its peak. The car is being pushed past its ability to maintain high-performance balance and will eventually break down. Do you really think you have a chance at winning the race this way?

Heck no! The smart thing to do would be to make a simple pit stop!

You have no chance of winning a race with this strategy. Those signals are all there for a reason, and a great driver pays attention to those signals and responds to them as needed. A horrible driver ignores the signals, believing he can push the car and win the race. Eventually the driver pushes the car too far, and it either breaks down or runs out of gas. Now the car is "dead" and unable to respond to any of the driver's commands. No matter how hard the driver pushes on the gas pedal, if there's no gas in the tank, there will be no response from the car.

This is what happens to your body when it's put under unneces-

A Simple Adrenal Test You Can Do at Home

Here's a simple test you can do at home to see how your adrenals are doing called the Orthostatic Hypotension Test. It's a test we run on every client who walks into Stark to get some clues as to how well their adrenals are doing. To complete the test you need a blood pressure cuff and a place to lie down flat on your back. Place the blood pressure cuff on your arm and lie comfortably, flat on your back, for 5 minutes. Take your blood pressure and record the systolic number (top number). Next come to a standing position and retake your blood pressure. Again record the systolic number (top number). See the chart below for results.

ORTHOSTATIC HYPOTENSION TEST RESULTS	
Systolic Change	*Possible Adrenal Finding*
Increases 6–10 mm/Hg	Healthy adrenal function
Increases 1–6 mm/Hg or does not change	Adrenals are under stress
Decreases 1–10 mm/Hg	Adrenals are struggling
Decreases more than 10 mm/Hg	Adrenals are exhausted

If your systolic number does not go up by 6–10 mm/Hg, you know you are in the Metabolic Breakdown Cycle, but if it drops more than 10 mm/Hg, you need to follow the guidelines in this chapter. You might not officially be there (you would need a 16-hour saliva cortisol DHEA lab to confirm this for sure), but it's pretty clear your adrenals have been overworked and are really struggling. It's time to give them some serious support.

sary stress. So many of us totally ignore our body's signals that something is wrong. We are determined to push through everything! You can't win in this game of life by ignoring the signals.

Your body is trying everything to force you to sleep, yet you keep slamming coffee and Red Bulls to push through! Your headache is screaming for water, yet you give it an aspirin!

Gentlemen, your body needs green vegetables to rise to the occasion, but your answer is Viagra to improve blood flow. Ladies, the fat accumulating around your hips and thighs is begging you to hit the stress-reduction button, yet you continue to do the opposite and keep grinding through workouts. When you choose to ignore the stress signals crying out from your body, forcing it to keep going, the adrenal glands eventually become overworked and start shutting down.

The HP complex will elevate the signaling, trying to get the lethargic adrenal glands to respond, but it too will eventually give out. Now, the overworked adrenal glands and HP complex are just like the run-down race car and no longer able to signal and respond.

If you are experiencing symptoms of adrenal burnout, your adrenal glands and the HP complex in your brain have been pushed too hard, too long. They can no longer keep up with the demands. The only answer is to make a pit stop and reset your metabolism.

How the Stark Naked 21-Day Reset and Lifestyle Repair Adrenal Burnout

Is it as simple as just following the 21-Day Reset to fix adrenal burnout?

I wish! You didn't reach this state overnight, and therefore you won't fix it overnight. You have been ignoring your body's signals for years; the fact is, adrenal burnout is a pretty extreme chronic state.

To resolve your adrenal burnout, follow the Phase 1 Reset and Phase 2 Optimized Nutrition Plan *and* change how you think about stress. The Reset and Optimized Nutrition Plan will help reduce the lifestyle stressors contributing to your burnout. To heal, you'll also need to address your mental or emotional stress. And that means *reducing* it in your life.

I know, it's a lot easier said than done. Rome wasn't built in a day.

It will take time, but like everything we've talked about so far, it will be worth it.

In Chapter 2 we discussed the Hulk response and used the example of people allowing their inner Hulk to be activated simply because they are stuck in traffic. There was no life-threatening situation, but how they perceived the situation and the thoughts that followed caused them to respond internally as if it were.

This type of response to stress only leads down the path to destruction—especially where your health is concerned. Remember, this is your time to *relax and conquer*!

How can you accomplish this?

If you really want to recover from adrenal burnout, you will need to take some time and make a list of mental and emotional triggers that bring out your inner Hulk. I know one of my inner-Hulk triggers is being late. I despise running late. I used to get very worked up when I was late for an appointment, especially if someone else was the cause of my tardiness. I still get worked up about this, but I've learned not to let my inner Hulk come out over it, because I now understand that I pay the price for that response.

Even so, there are times that test me. As a guy who grew up in the rains of Oregon, I hate how life in Southern California comes to a screeching halt with the slightest drizzle. The roads become gridlocked, and everyone is afraid to drive. If I have to drop my kids off at school in the morning, which is usually a major treat for me, and then get to a meeting with a client, it becomes a real challenge in the rain. I will feel my inner Hulk emerging, but I try my hardest to fight it, as I inch my way through the drop-off lane, watching the clock, knowing it's going to be close whether I'll make my meeting on time or not.

Once you've made your list of triggers, you will want to avoid those situations until you've learned to control them. If you find yourself experiencing the trigger, you will need to remind yourself that it's not a life-or-death scenario. No matter what, everything will be okay. You may have to practice deep breathing until you feel calm and in control. A mentor of mine George Ryan puts it nicely: "Take a walk on the beach in your mind for a few minutes," meaning find a calm place in your mind until you're at peace. Do whatever it takes to either avoid those stress triggers or keep yourself calm whenever you're experiencing them.

You will also want to take up some type of meditation to calm your inner Hulk. Meditation is one of the greatest tools available to high performers. There is a reason people like Oprah, Richard Branson, and Tony Robbins are constantly recommending meditation. It's a major competitive advantage for greatness. But if you are anything like me, when I close my eyes and try to think about nothing, I literally think about everything. It's far from relaxing, because I just end up getting frustrated. A couple of smartphone apps that I really like to use to help me reach a meditative state are *Calm* and *Headspace*. Find what works for you and use it regularly.

Last, you need to focus on two things we have yet to talk about—your recovery and sleep. Sleep is such a critical component in your

Keep Calm!

My favorite app for keeping my inner Hulk under control is *Calm.* It progressively relaxes your body until you hit a deeply calm and relaxed state. I use this app two or three times a day, because it keeps my stress under control and helps me feel my best.

Another app I really like is *Headspace.* I love to use this app before I speak, as it centers me and calms my mind, making me a much better speaker.

I also recommend any type of mindset training that helps you cope with stressful situations. I have included a few of my favorites in the Resource Guide.

When you combine a bulletproof mindset with a reset, high-performing metabolism, you can accomplish things beyond your greatest dreams!

reset, especially if you have hit the wall. Later, in Chapter 8, I am going to explain why it's so important and give you my best strategies for improving it. You will learn in greater detail why I believe sleep is the fountain of youth, the wellspring of your sex hormones, and the source of your energy and creativity.

Sleep is your secret weapon and greatest asset to recovering from adrenal burnout. Just following the Stark Naked 21-Day Metabolic Reset alone without committing to great sleep at this stage of the breakdown cycle will leave you with subpar results. Remember, you have to start making deposits back into your overdrawn energy account. This means you'll have to commit to 7 to 9 hours of quality sleep. If your schedule doesn't allow for that kind of time, you need to do some negotiating elsewhere. Real rejuvenation happens in sleep, and depriving yourself of sleep is one of the reasons you have ended up feeling this way. Everyone experiencing adrenal-burnout symptoms has cheated sleep at some point in their life.

Guess what? You can't win this game of life if you are cheating sleep. Period!

Plain and simple, either make some room for it or get ready to spend the remainder of your life being unproductive and feeling miserable. It's your call. I have yet to meet someone who complains about the quality of work, level of production, and general improvement in life as a result of sleeping more.

I have a confession to make. I have been known to be a little hardheaded from time to time. Sometimes it takes reliving pain a few times before I truly learn my lesson. I have lived the adrenal burnout nightmare twice in my life. The Stark Naked 21-Day Metabolic Reset pulled me out of my last adrenal-burnout state, and the Phase 2 Optimized Nutrition Plan has kept me living a beautiful life that is busier than ever.

Life is so much better when you live it with boundless energy. I want you to experience that more than anything! This plan is truly made for resurrecting those who find themselves in this ugly world known as adrenal burnout, and it's there to change trajectory for those of you who haven't hit rock bottom yet, but are on a collision course toward it. It will take some commitment and effort on your part to resuscitate yourself, but trust me you will learn to love giving back to yourself. It's okay to love yourself every day! In my opinion, it's your duty!

When you choose to ignore the stress signals crying out from your body, forcing it to keep going, the adrenal glands eventually become overworked and start shutting down. To resolve your adrenal burnout, follow the Phase 1 Reset and Phase 2 Optimized Nutrition Plan, reduce your mental/emotional stress, and prioritize sleep.

Jeff, ex-Navy SEAL, currently with Search and Rescue California
Age forty-eight

▶ *Jeff was referred to me because he was experiencing extreme lethargy. Just getting out of bed was a chore! As an ex-Navy SEAL, he found that lack of energy tough to take. He was tired of feeling and looking worn out and wanted answers. Jeff was once the physical and mental specimen every man dreams of being, but now he found himself far from the picture of the man he once was. He just couldn't understand why he was always so tired. No amount of sleep seemed to help him feel better. More didn't seem to solve his problem, and less just made it worse.*

His daily exercise regime with his current tactical team had no positive effect on how he looked or felt either. Usually, exercise gave him some kind of boost. But now it only made him drag more. Jeff really began to notice the effects of extreme fatigue when he was sent out on calls searching for lost hikers. Mountainous terrain that was once easy for him was now extremely challenging and taxing.

Despite eating the same as he always had, Jeff was slowly

gaining weight, getting fatter in areas that had never been an issue. As the days went on it, it took everything in him to just survive his workouts.

After running the Orthostatic Hypotension Test on Jeff to determine if he was suffering from adrenal burnout, my hunch proved right. His systolic number dropped 30 points when he stood up. Jeff was clearly experiencing adrenal burnout and needed to be rejuvenated.

As a Navy SEAL, this man possessed more mental willpower than you or I could imagine, yet his extreme willpower and drive were of no avail. His intense drive to force change was only creating negative change, which left him feeling frustrated and angry.

I love working with guys like Jeff, because I get to be the brakes, not the gas pedal. Unmotivated people need a cheerleader to push their gas pedal and get them off the couch to exercise; high performers like Jeff need a brakeman—someone to help them pull the reigns back and allow the body to recover from all of the demands placed on it over the years. Most high achievers just need a great strategy to reset and renew their systems to experience incredible results.

During our first meeting Jeff weighed in at 186 pounds with 16 percent body fat. His first goal was to get his energy and ambition back in life. His second goal was to get his Navy SEAL body back. Following the initial Stark Naked 21-Day Metabolic Reset, Jeff focused on recovering from an extremely high-stress lifestyle. He was amazed by his rejuvenated energy and drive. Within the first couple of weeks, Jeff actually looked forward to getting out of bed and enjoyed challenging himself in the gym again. His weight dropped to 180 pounds and his body fat reduced to 12.5 percent. Four months later, his weight held steady at 175 pounds, and his body fat percentage got back to where it was during his SEAL days at 9 percent.

▶ PART THREE

THE STARK
NAKED
LIFESTYLE
FOR SUCCESS

7

Breaking Bad

Clarifying Nutritional Confusion

I F COUNTING CALORIES was the gold-standard way to get the best weight-loss results, I would not have written this book. Frankly, I'd likely be out of a job. I never learned how to count calories. It's not that I can't count or add. I surely can—unless you're doing reps in my gym! In which case, ten is never really just ten. But that's another story. However, when it comes to counting calories, well, I've never subscribed to that theory.

My original journey in the fitness realm started just as a personal trainer and strength coach. I didn't start to focus on nutrition until the late 1990s. When I started working at a high-end gym in 1998 that had a nutritionist on staff, I did what all the smart trainers did. I sent my clients to the nutritionist to enhance their results. At least that was the promise I was sold by the owner of the gym, and like my clients I bought into the better-diet-equals-better-results pitch.

Every diet that my clients received early on was focused solely on calories. I watched as each of my clients started to feel miserable, losing strength and stamina in the process. Worse, their body fat rarely came down. In fact, for many it starting going up. At the time, my uneducated answer was to train harder, do more reps, and eat less.

Hey, it was all about calories, and if they were eating too many calories, I was going to make up for it by having them expend more calories. This approach only left my clients feeling exhausted and frustrated.

The nutritionists told me it was my clients' fault. Their lack of results was due to overeating and lying in their food journals. How annoying was that?

My clients and I were at our wits' end. Something had to give, so I changed the plan. I started experimenting.

The first thing I did was to meet with the top three nutrition experts in my area and have them design nutrition programs for me. At the time all three focused on calories. I knew that wasn't going to work. Been there, done that. Still, I gave all three the same diet and exercise outline I was following, and I got three totally different answers for my calorie needs. I chose the one I felt was the best fit for me and the results were staggering. I put on 5 percent body fat in the first six weeks! I was furious! My goal was to drop body fat, not add it!

At my follow-up meeting, the grave conclusion was that it was my fault, I was lying about what I said I ate, and I needed to be more honest about everything I was eating. I didn't take this criticism well, as I tend to go above and beyond with my efforts. I was always told by coaches growing up that I was incredibility coachable. In fact, my coaches had to choose wisely what they asked of me, because I applied it exactly as requested. I was obsessed with getting results.

So in this case I had followed the diet outline perfectly and to the letter. Needless to say, I quickly abandoned that low-calorie, fat-gaining trap and started my own journey, which has led me to acquire knowledge and strategies over the years that are responsible for the success of this program.

Do High Achievers Really Overeat?

I have reviewed thousands of high achievers' diets over the years, including those of pro athletes, tactical athletes, CEOs, homemakers, entrepreneurs, high-school athletes, CrossFit athletes, and busy executives, and the one commonality among all of them is that the majority undereat. Their metabolisms are paying the price for eating too little, which is what makes them feel and look miserable. It's amazing how many women are losing their hair and have zero sex drive from caloric deprivation. Yet if you ask them what strategies they are using to change their outcome, they will say, "I know I eat too much, so I am watching my calories."

I am not naive, nor am I saying calories are of zero importance. If you weigh 120 pounds and eat 8,000 calories a day you will gain weight. However, I hardly ever meet anyone who is actually, genuinely overeating. Most of us are too busy to overeat. The only issue with calories for most high achievers is that they need to consume more! Scary thought, but it's the truth.

I've learned one very important fact: *no matter how few calories you eat, you will never succeed by depriving your metabolism of what it needs.* Doing this is a recipe for metabolic disaster.

There are far too many nutritional "rules" that cause confusion and hold us back from living our healthiest lives.

One Size Does Not Fit All

In Chapter 1, I listed several variations of popular diets and nutritional plans that most of you have either heard of or likely tried at one time or another. From these you can get some idea of what has gotten you to this broken state. Since the 1960s, research has been dominated by two conflicting observations. First, we are under the misguided impression that the so-called experts know how to eat healthy and maintain a healthy weight. Some do, some don't. Second, the obesity rate has nearly tripled since the 1960s, which suggests that something about these dieting approaches isn't working.

There have been tens of thousands of diet books and articles on health and nutrition over the years offering all sorts of plans promising all sorts of ideas, hypothesis, research, knowledge, science, and data to show "their" ideas work. Most experts believe their program is the be-all and end-all answer for every individual alive.

Is there one perfect program that works for everyone? I haven't found one yet. Sure, some are better than others. And some, well, I am not a fan of at all. I believe my plan is better than most, because it's a manageable lifestyle that can be maintained, but I will concede it too isn't perfect for everyone.

When it comes to nutritional health and wellness, my philosophy is pretty simple. *Find the foods or dietary patterns that help you in your pursuit of a long and healthy life.*

I have learned many strategies from various medical experts that have been incorporated into the Stark Naked 21-Day Metabolic Reset to help make sure you discover the benefits of true healthy living and maintain this new lifestyle. I get it. You don't have the time to be sick and rundown. None of us do. That's why I've taken the guesswork out of it for you.

I've also incorporated some great strategies learned over the years from fat-loss experts, because I believe having a lower body fat is a competitive advantage in all areas of high performance, except perhaps in Sumo wrestling. The remainder of the strategies you'll experience throughout this program have come from trial and error—lots of trial and error. These are strategies that have worked for my clients and for me.

Remember, what got you here won't get you there.

Busting the Six Nutritional "Rules" Holding You Back

There are six main nutritional "rules" that cause my clients the greatest amount of confusion and hold them back from living their healthiest lives. For many, these rules are set in stone. Yet few people I train have ever taken the time to research the validity of these so-called rules or why they should abide by them in the first place. As a result, most people believe and therefore trust that if they want to stay fit and healthy, these are the key things they're supposed to do, and they therefore dutifully follow along.

I've got news for you. These so-called rules are really nothing more than urban myths.

For example, you may believe it is necessary to eat five or six small meals a day to get your metabolism charged and live in an optimal state. Or you may believe you can't eat carbs—at all. Or, if you do eat carbs, you may believe you can't eat them at night.

Guess what?

Not one of those is true!

Warning: Not only am I going to challenge these so-called rules of successful nutrition; I am going to ask you to break them!

I know what you're thinking. "Say, what? Break the rules? No way! I can't do that! If I do, my metabolism will slow down, and I will get fat."

Stop it! Stop right now. Let's be honest with ourselves. If you're reading this book, your metabolism is far from optimal. Something has got to change! Maybe it's one of your precious nutritional rules!

I am only challenging you to try the Reset for 21 days. Then decide for yourself.

Here are the six nutritional rules *you* are going to break *now* to ensure your success.

Nutritional Rule #1: You must eat five to six meals a day to keep your metabolism at its peak and prevent you from going into starvation mode.

How many of you believe this one?

Okay, I will admit that I followed this advice for the longest time. As a good trainer, I even passed this knowledge on to my clients. "You must eat every 2 to 3 hours, or you'll risk your metabolism slowing and your body going into starvation mode," I'd preach.

Here's the truth. If this rule were an undeniable fact, science would back it up as the best way to eat. Well, it doesn't.

Science continuously shows no benefit from this rule, which makes this a myth. It is true that digesting a meal raises metabolism slightly, a phenomenon known as the thermic effect of food. However, it is the total amount of food consumed that determines the amount of energy expended during digestion. Eating three meals of 800 calories will cause the same thermic effect as eating six meals of 400 calories. There is literally no difference.

There is no nutritional benefit to eating smaller meals more often. Numerous studies are now showing it to actually underperform in comparison with larger, less frequent meals. A study published in the *International Journal of Obesity and Metabolic Related Disorders* put this to the test. All subjects ate the same number of calories, but they were divided up into different meal frequencies: six meals a day, two large meals a day, or fasting for breakfast. Zero benefit was found for higher-frequency meal consumption. There was no significant effect on metabolic rate or total fat lost by eating more often, even though the nutritional world has told us the opposite.

In 2012, a study published by Maastricht University Medical Center compared high-frequency meals with low-frequency meals, and the results were the opposite of what was expected. Resting metabolic rate (RMR) was higher in the low-frequency meal group, meaning the subjects' metabolism was more elevated. The study also found appetite control was better in the low-frequency meal group.

How can that be? What about blood sugar? Aren't small meals more often supposed to be better for blood-sugar control? Aren't we supposed to eat meals every 2 to 3 hours to control our blood sugar and keep our appetite under control?

According to this study, the low-frequency eating *reduced* overall glucose levels during the day, indicating glycemic improvements. These are just two of the many studies that have found that increased meal frequency creates no benefit to your metabolism and often decreases your ability to lose weight.

Perhaps you're wondering, "Okay, but what about my muscle mass. If I don't eat every 2 to 3 hours I will go into starvation mode, and my muscles will start to feed off themselves, right? I can't risk losing muscle mass, Brad."

I totally agree that muscle mass is critical. I even believe maintaining muscle mass is a great predictor of longevity. But let's take a look at an interesting study that may change your mind.

The *British Journal of Nutrition* reported a study on how the body and metabolism respond to fasting for durations of 12, 36, and 72 hours. If 2 to 3 hours is all it takes to go into starvation mode, then after 12 hours people should be crushed. By 72 hours they should be absolutely destroyed, right?

Wrong! At the 12- and 36-hour marks, the researchers found enhanced metabolisms, not sluggish ones. The starvation mode switch does exist, but it didn't kick in with the people in this study until the 72-hour mark. Rule busted.

Nutritional Rule #2: Always eat carbohydrates in the morning.

We've all heard this: eat carbohydrates early in the day for good energy and so you will easily burn them off with regular daily activity.

As a high achiever, you likely rely on having a lot of energy and a sharp, focused brain. If you lack energy or your brain is not in the game, your performance will suffer greatly. If carbohydrates were the answer for enhanced energy and performance, you would eat carbs with every meal, right? Logic would say that by doing so, you'd always have great energy and great focus, but we hardly find that to be the case at Stark. Most people we test and work with experience the opposite effect when eating carbs. They complain of feeling lethargic and sleepy after eating carbs. If you don't believe me, join me for a corporate speaking engagement following a pasta lunch. Most people want to take a nap—and some do, heads bobbing and eyes rolling trying to stay awake. It isn't my topic! What they need is some protein.

I remember game days back in high school. Our coach always encouraged the team to eat huge carb-loading meals before football and basketball games. He said the carbs were supposed to give us an energy edge. The problem was that the majority of my teammates and I would fall asleep on the bus ride to the big game from all of those heavy carbs! The last thing we wanted to do when we arrived at our destination was to play a game—let alone win! We could have been much better athletes if our coach understood the impact of all those carbs on his team.

The hormonal response to carbohydrates causes a rise and fall of insulin, which makes you tired. The rise in insulin triggers the brain to release serotonin, a neurotransmitter that calms and relaxes the brain. It's why Thanksgiving is so great at inducing your food coma. It's not so much the tryptophan in the turkey (that does help a bit), but the carbs you eat with the turkey that cause the rise in insulin and release of serotonin.

The reality is, carb loading before the big game or important match isn't good for any athlete. It was a misunderstood myth everyone bought into back then. Now that I am a coach and trainer, I want my competitive athletes showing up for their competitions supercharged, on fire, wanting nothing more than to be engaged in their competition, not dreaming of a nap. You can bet I am not feeding them carbs before the big event we spend so much time training for!

If your goal is to have a lot of energy, to be more focused and highly driven, then you need to *avoid carbs early in the day*. The Stark Naked

21-Day Metabolic Reset is built to support this concept by providing you with foods early in the day that keep insulin at bay and the brain turned on—not shutting down.

The ideal foods for great energy and brain power are protein and fat. They don't create the major spike in insulin that carbohydrates do, therefore keeping the brain from shutting down. Eating protein and fats early in the day is the foundation of true high-performance nutrition. Interestingly, you will notice in Phase 1 that you are not asked to eat these foods for breakfast. Why?

Detoxing your liver is a major focus at the start of the plan. If your liver is sluggish and you eat protein and fats too early in the day, it can make you nauseous. The liver is required to help break down the proteins and fats, so you need it humming along and not behind on its duty to get the most out of the protein and fat intake.

Nutritional Rule #3: Eating carbohydrates at night will make you fat.

Okay, great. So now you understand the reason you shouldn't eat carbs in the morning. But I know what you're thinking. "There's no way I am eating carbs at night! It will make me fat!"

I get it. We all want to look great. I want to look great as well, but this whole idea that eating carbs at night will make us fat is far from verified in the world of science. Yes, during the first half of sleep there is a dip in energy usage, but during the second half of sleep, in the REM cycles, energy expenditure takes off again. Believing that energy expenditure is so low during sleep that carbs will make you fat is ludicrous. Science is beginning to back the notion that eating carbs at night will not only make you lose more weight than spreading carbs throughout the day, but it will also enhance the quality of your sleep. It's a two-for-one special!

In 2011, a group of Israeli scientists found that those who ate 80 percent or more of their carbohydrate intake starting at dinner over the course of six months not only lost more weight and body fat, but also had fewer issues with hunger during the day. Why wouldn't you want those kinds of benefits from your nutrition?

Research has also shown that eating a meal at night with carbs in it helps induce sleep. It enhances pathways in our body that make us sleepy, whereas protein blocks those pathways making you feel more awake. Now, understand that this isn't the green light to start eating a bunch of junk carbohydrates before bed. High-sugar carbs will make you crash quickly, but they will disrupt overall sleep.

The research is clear. A higher-protein diet during the day and whole-food carbs like sweet potatoes at night is the key to success. Just follow the exact outline of the 21-Day Reset, and you will benefit from all this great cutting-edge research without having to think about it.

This rule is by far the hardest of the six biggies to get my clients to break. Everyone I work with believes that eating carbs is bad, so getting my clients to eat carbs at night is one of my greatest challenges. But when they finally give in and trust in the process and the plan, the results speak for themselves. The weight loss and improved sleep are enough to turn any doubter into a believer.

Still don't buy into it? Try it for 21 days. If you're not completely convinced, go back to your old ways. You've got nothing to lose, and everything to gain. I'll stake my name and reputation on it!

Nutritional Rule #4: Removing foods like dairy and gluten (wheat) is dangerous and will lead to nutrient deficiencies.

This rule is one of my favorites to debunk.

Here's an interesting fact. Every single one of us is walking around with multiple nutrient deficiencies that are caused either by genetic issues, poor digestion, lack of nutrients in the soil our foods were grown in, or simple lack of consumption. You definitely are and, despite my knowledge and awareness, I am too.

The value of proper nutritional balance is not very important to most people, but our bodies were designed to function at the highest level by absorbing vitamins and minerals from the food we eat. A nutritional deficiency occurs when the body doesn't absorb the necessary amount of a nutrient. Calcium, vitamin D, iron, potassium, vitamin B_{12}, magnesium, and folate deficiencies make it tough for your body to run optimally and can be the source of symptoms like fatigue, hair loss, muscle cramps, skin issues, digestion issues, stunted or defective bone growth, and even dementia, just to name a few. On a cellular level, nutrient deficiencies can impact bodily functions including water balance, enzyme function, nerve signaling, and metabolism.

In the past I've experienced numbness in my hands at night while I sleep. For me this was caused by B_{12} deficiency with a known genetic basis. Vitamin B_{12} not only helps with healthy nerve cells; it is also involved in red-blood-cell production, aids in the production of DNA, and helps make neurotransmitters in the brain. Interestingly, although my vitamin deficiency is genetic, vitamin B_{12} deficiency is becoming much more common today, especially among vegans and people who've had weight-loss surgery. The symptoms of B_{12} deficiency include numbness in the legs, hands, or feet; problems with walking and balance; anemia; fatigue; weakness; depression; a swollen, inflamed tongue; memory loss; paranoia; and hallucinations. If you have any of these symptoms, you can get vitamin B_{12} from eating more fish, eggs, and poultry.

Okay, you're probably confused. So let me explain.

If these nutrients are so important, why would I remove foods that would put anyone at risk for increasing their deficiencies? Good question!

First, the only reason dairy and gluten are of concern is because the typical American diet is so poor and devoid of nutrients that dairy and gluten-containing grains, such as wheat, barley, and rye, are often the only sources of nutrients at all. The reality is that nutrients are hidden in our vegetables and fruits, and those are what most people tend to have the hardest time eating.

"Eat your fruits and vegetables." We've heard that all our lives,

OTHER COMMON NUTRIENT DEFICIENCIES		
Nutrient	Where It's Found (Stark Approved)	Deficiency Symptoms
Vitamin B$_2$	Lamb, oily fish (mackerel), eggs, spinach, asparagus, collard greens, mushrooms	Anemia, cataracts, poor thyroid function, fatigue, bloodshot eyes, chapped lips, sore tongue and lips
Folate	Spinach, asparagus, avocados, mango, oranges	Anemia, poor immune function, fatigue, insomnia, elevated homocysteine
Zinc	Poultry, seafood, lamb, wild game meat, spinach, pomegranates, blackberries	Hair loss, diarrhea, impotence, loss of appetite, loss of taste, weight loss, slow wound healing, mental lethargy
Magnesium	Dark leafy green vegetables (spinach), avocados, fish, blackberries, raspberries	Nausea, vomiting, muscle cramps or twitching, insomnia, anxiety, restlessness, irritability
Vitamin D	Sunlight, egg yolks, fish	Osteoporosis, low calcium absorption, depression, bone ache, head sweating

right? Most of you probably know they decrease your risk of diseases like cancer and yet so few focus on eating those foods that benefit you most. If you are really worried about nutrient deficiencies, then step up and eat your fruits and vegetables. If you follow my program, like it or not, you will!

By increasing your consumption of these foods, you will avoid any nutrient deficiencies that might occur because foods such as dairy and gluten are no longer in your diet. We want dairy, gluten, and all of the other foods that commonly trigger inflammation removed for all of the reasons we explored in Chapter 4. That inflammation response is not worth the pathetic batch of nutrients you are getting from dairy and gluten, nutrients that you could be getting in abundance from your fruits and vegetables without the adverse reaction. This is killing two birds with one stone. Remove the irritants and enhance your uptake of nutrients. It's so simple!

Nutritional Rule #5: You have to restrict calories for weight-loss success.

At the very beginning of this chapter I stated that I don't agree with the low-calorie approach, but I really want to drive this point home, because so many people obsess about this so-called rule. In my opinion, there are much deeper and more important reasons holding you back than eating too many calories. According to Gary Taubes, who wrote the book *Why We Get Fat: And What to Do About It*, in 1878 the German nutritionist Max Rubner crafted what he called the "isodynamic law." This law claimed that the basis of nutrition is simply the exchange of energy, spawning the belief that "a calorie is a calorie." This means that no matter what the source of a calorie (fat, protein, or carb), the energy extracted from it or the work necessary to burn it is the same.

For over a hundred years science has been drilling this idea into us. Consume fewer calories than you burn, and you will lose weight. Consume more, and the number on the scale will increase. If you are gaining weight, you are simply eating too many calories. Therefore, the only solution is to eat less or exercise more. Get serious about your weight and do both.

Here's how this theory works. A pound of fat is 3,500 calories. If you eat 500 calories less than you burn every day, then after a week (7 × 500 = 3,500) you will have lost a pound of fat.

Wow! I wish it were that easy. If that were the case, we'd all be walking around skinny and happy, and I'd be unemployed.

I'm always amazed by the variations in the way people approach this simple calorie-restriction idea. I remember speaking with one woman a few years ago whose trainer had her exercising twice a day, 7 days a week. He was only allowing her to eat 800 calories a day, assuring her it didn't matter what foods made up those 800 calories, claiming it could be birthday cake or Ring Dings; as long as she stayed at 800 calories, she would see results. Theoretically, she was burning more calories than she was consuming, so she should have gotten skinny overnight, yet the exact opposite happened. In her case, calorie deprivation backfired. The number on the scale went up from unwanted fat accumulation around her hips and thighs. How in the world could that happen when she was in extreme calorie deprivation?

Because calorie restriction for weight loss is a myth and not supported by science. In 2004, a study in the *Journal of Nutrition and Metabolism* divided overweight individuals into two groups. One group was fed a high-protein diet, and the other was given a high-carbohydrate diet. The high-carbohydrate group was fed an average of 300 fewer calories a day. At first glance, the study appeared straightforward. According to the "a calorie is a calorie" model, the lower-calorie intake group should have lost more weight, but the exact opposite happened. The higher-calorie, high-protein group ended up losing more weight and more fat in the study.

What? How can that be? Why did the high-protein group lose more weight, even though they consumed more calories? There are a few reasons.

First, food affects hormones. In this study carbohydrates triggered the release of insulin telling the body to store energy, not burn it. Second, the amount of energy the body uses to break down, assimilate, and absorb protein is much greater than what the body uses to break down carbohydrates.

The third and final possible reason the high-protein group may have lost more weight is the fact that protein consumption creates more satiety. That may not have been the case in this study if everything eaten was carefully monitored, but in real life it is easier to overeat on a high-carbohydrate diet. This study shows it's more important to focus on what you eat rather than how much.

So if it's not all about the calories, what causes us to put on weight?

The human metabolism is so complex. There are so many variables that can cause weight gain. The Stark Naked 21-Day Metabolic Reset deals with the three major causes of fat gain for high achievers—*stress* from a high-achieving lifestyle, *toxicity,* and *food-driven inflammation.* You can reduce your calories as much as you want, but if your metabolism is broken, the calorie pursuit is pointless and just fuels fat gain.

A few years back I was working with an NFL lineman who quickly needed to lose 25 pounds. This man weighed 372 pounds. A team was interested in him, but would only sign him if he could get his weight down to 350 pounds. Strangely, he was only eating 2,400 calories a day, not a lot for a guy that size. My initial comment was "You are starving yourself! My eleven-year-old eats more than you do!"

He told me that two weeks prior to our conversation the food delivery company he was using increased his calories from 2,400 to 2,800 calories a day, and his weight increased from 360 to 372 pounds. He was forced to return to 2,400 calories, as that was all he could eat without gaining weight. My client was exercising hard to try to lose the weight, but wasn't getting any result. He felt horrible, had no energy, and was not gaining any strength in the gym. He definitely wasn't lying to me about what he was eating. It's amazing how honest people are when specific changes in their bodies equal a bigger bank account!

Don't believe me? Just watch an episode of *The Biggest Loser.*

You become very honest and are willing to do anything for success. Since cutting calories was not an option, I had to make a quick decision. I remembered my client mentioning he was having weird cravings for things like dairy and wheat bread. That's when it occurred to me that there was something else going on. I immediately called the food delivery company he used for all of his meals and asked them to remove all the common foods that people have sensitivities to, those that we remove in Phase 1 of the Reset.

The result? Within eight weeks he was down to 340 pounds!

"I don't understand this," he said. "I have more energy than I have had in years! My strength in the gym is unreal! I haven't weighed this little since high school, and I am eating more calories! I should feel miserable right now from the effort and sacrifice to reach this weight, but I feel great! I have always been made to feel it was my fault, like I wasn't trying hard enough or I was lying to them on my low-calorie programs. No one believed me except you."

The sincerity in his words was the best part of our success. I simply replied, "We found the root cause of your broken metabolism, food-driven inflammation, and repaired it."

Nutritional Rule #6: Caving in to cravings is just a lack of willpower. Suck it up!

When it comes to cravings, a lot of my clients are very shy when talking to me about their habits. They see their hankerings for midnight snacks and novel food combinations as strange and weak.

Allow me to be the bearer of some good news. Cravings are a real issue in today's society. There are all kinds of theories behind cravings.

Some claim they are merely a given and need to be controlled by willpower, while others say the food industry discovers our addiction mechanisms and preys on them. When a potato-chip manufacturer says, "You can't eat just one . . . ," believe it.

After my first food sensitivity test was done, I discovered that the foods on my sensitivity list were the same foods I often found myself craving—a lot. This piqued my curiosity, especially because I found it really hard to break my addiction to those foods I was sensitive to—specifically maple syrup and dairy products. I wasn't sure how I would prove it, but I was certain there was a connection.

Every Friday, my high-carb cheat meal (which you will learn more about in Phase 2, the Optimized Nutrition Plan) was pancakes or waffles with a *ton* of maple syrup and ice cream. I loved the flavor combination of that dessert. However, once I ate it on Friday, I found myself having nearly uncontrollable cravings for it during the following week. It took every ounce of willpower I had not to give in to my desire for that dessert until the following Friday.

However, one Friday I ate those same foods, and my throat started to close up. The severe reaction almost choked me to death. Now, you might have thought this experience would have been scary enough to keep me from ever eating that dessert again—but it wasn't. My cravings were so strong that I continued with my Friday-night habit despite knowing it could kill me.

Originally, I thought it must be the gluten in the pancakes, until one weekend I was visiting my parents with my daughter and my mom made us gluten-free pancakes. Thinking I was in the clear, I poured maple syrup over the top and began to eat. Again my throat closed up, but this time it was the worst experience I'd ever had. And this time, it took place in front of my daughter.

Okay, now I began to worry I might be sensitive to all carbs. That breakfast was the tipping point that pushed me to have my sensitivity test done. Lo and behold it wasn't the gluten. It was the maple syrup and cow's milk that was roughing me up. Ta-dah!

I immediately went to IHOP and devoured a huge plate of pancakes with blueberry syrup—not maple—followed by dairy-free ice cream. Guess what? No choking response.

As I ran more and more of these tests, it suddenly became very clear to me that people actually crave the foods they are most likely to be sensitive to. My hypothesis gets proven with every client MRT that comes back. The foods my clients crave the most usually appear in their red zone—meaning these are the foods they shouldn't eat, because they trigger an intense inflammation response and do the greatest harm.

It is not clear why we often crave foods to which we are sensitive, but several theories have been proposed. Some researchers suggest that our bodies can become addicted to the chemical messengers, such as histamine or cortisol, that are secreted by immune cells in response to allergens in the body. It is hypothesized that, although eating foods to which you are allergic can cause a rash or sneezing, the body also may experience a soothing response from the presence of the chemical messengers, increasing the desire to eat more of that food.

Another theory proposed by a well-known immunologist is based on the science of how antibodies (a protein used by the immune system to identify and neutralize foreign objects) and antigens (unique parts of the foreign object) connect (bind) to each other. Antibodies can bind to more than one site on an allergen in the food; therefore, when there are very few antigens but a large number of antibodies present, the antibodies will become cross-linked and make large complexes. It is theorized that these large complexes can cause an increase in symptoms.

In this theory symptoms are caused by the large number of antibodies in relation to the number of antigens rather than being caused by the number of antigens. In fact, it is suggested that if you eat more of the antigen, you can decrease the number of antibody complexes by allowing each antibody to bind to an antigen rather than forming the large complexes, thereby reducing the number of symptoms. Normal metabolism works to remove the food antigens, and as the ratio of antibodies to antigens begins to rise, symptoms will begin to increase. Craving and addiction to food may be the result of the body's attempt to increase the number of antigens present and prevent the formation of the large antibody complexes that are associated with an increased number of symptoms.

Succumbing to food cravings to help alleviate symptoms provides short-term relief. The cravings and symptoms will return. This yo-yo effect is believed by some allergy specialists to be the reason why people who stop eating the foods to which they are allergic first go through several days when they feel worse before they start feeling much better.

The important thing to remember is that *you don't know how bad you're feeling until you eliminate the cause of your stress.* You have learned to live and, worse, accept living with feeling bad. Once you cleanse your body of the toxins that are causing you to feel your worst, you will appreciate what it feels like to be back at your best.

Breaking the Rules Is Fun!

Breaking the "rules" of nutrition can be scary and tough. One of the best strategies I have seen work is to complete the Stark Naked 21-Day Metabolic Reset with a community of family and friends. If you are married, do whatever it takes to get your spouse to join you on the Reset. Support, especially during the first week, is critical and leads to incredible long-term success. There's great power in numbers.

Craig and Cherisse Smyser are a couple in their early forties from Texas who went on the Stark Naked 21-Day Reset with Tom Ferry's original inner-circle real-estate group. Their results have been nothing short of life-changing. Here is their story, told by Cherisse:

About five years ago, I was working out in a gym 1 to 2 hours a day, 6 days a week, and I was in great shape, the best shape of my life. Then we moved back to Texas, and I found work as a preschool teacher. I stopped working out, and over the course of four years I gained about 35 pounds. Finally, I was able to go back to a gym, and although the weight came off a little (at the most, 10 pounds), it always came back on, even when I thought I was eating "right." I think my metabolism just kept my body at this new weight no matter what I did. Recently, I even tried Plexus Slim on a recommendation from friends. Nope. Nothing happened after four months using their pink drink.

Then my husband mentioned your Reset challenge, and we decided to do it as a couple. Craig ended up losing 10 pounds, and I shed 15! In three weeks! I feel amazing, and I'm looking forward to getting rid of another 20 pounds to get back down to the low 160s (I'm 5 foot 11). We are following Phase 2 and having no problems staying on it. And, although we look forward to that 7th-day high-carb meal, we don't feel like we need it. In addition, I have lost a total of 9 inches: 2 off my waist, 2½ off my hips, 1½ off my bust, 1 inch off each thigh, and ½ inch off each upper arm. And that's just in three weeks! Thank you for coming up with this program! It is finally something that my body responds to, and I feel so healthy. I love sugar, but I hardly even think about it anymore. I just didn't think that was possible!

One year later I received a follow-up e-mail from Cherisse. She and her husband were each down 30 pounds and loving life. This program is not a short-term fad diet. It's a life-changing alteration in lifestyle.

Breaking the rules can be fun, and oftentimes it takes a willingness to break the rules to find a pathway to success. Following the so-called nutritional rules is holding so many of you back. For the next 21 days I am going to ask you to put on a brave face and go rogue. Take a leap of faith with me and break the rules. You know as well as I do something has to change! What are you waiting for?

It's good to follow all the rules when you're young,
so you have the strength to break them when you're old.

—MARK TWAIN

I've broken all of the erroneous nutritional rules for you during your 21-Day Reset. The eleven fundamentals of the Stark Naked 21-Day Metabolic Reset (see page 204) help you to avoid the pitfalls of these so-called rules that are really holding you back.

9. Maximize protein and vegetable intake.
10. Follow carbohydrate and fat servings exactly.
11. Stick to three meals a day.

8

Sleep

Your Ultimate Ally

ONE OF THE FONDEST MEMORIES I have with my daughter, Isabel, was the first time she experienced the clear night sky at my parents' home in Oregon. She was just three years old and was mesmerized by how the bright stars lit up the night sky. Living in Southern California, she had never experienced anything quite like it. I had so much fun showing her the different constellations I grew up exploring as a young boy, like Orion's Belt and the Big Dipper. As we shared this father-daughter moment together, something extraordinary happened. Isabel got to see her first shooting star—and I was there to share in her excitement.

I grew up taking for granted the clear night skies of my home state. I suppose most of us don't appreciate what we have when we are kids until we are much older and can see those simple things through our children's eyes. As I think back, I vividly remember one night sleeping under the stars at summer camp. Like my daughter, I was enamored by the countless shooting stars I saw. I am quite certain I saw more shooting stars on that single night in Oregon than most people see in a lifetime.

It's not that the stars aren't as bright as ever—it's just that most people live in places where they will never see them unless they drive hours away. The city lights in most metropolitan cities at night are now so bright, they literally wipe out our ability to see the vastness of stars above us. According to the Tucson-based International Dark-Sky Association (IDA), the sky glow of Los Angeles is visible from an airplane two hundred miles away.

Thomas Edison and his invention of the lightbulb dramatically improved many areas of our lives. It also came with a cost. One of the biggest is the impact light has had on sleep.

I attended my first live fitness seminar in 2007 with world-renowned strength coach Charles Poliquin in Chicago. Charles was someone I had fanatically studied throughout high school and college. I read every article he ever wrote. Every month I'd rip through my new edition of *Muscle Media 2000* magazine looking for his next great tip to help make me bigger and stronger. So when I was able to attend this seminar and see him up close and personal, I was so jazzed to finally have the chance to spend 5 days learning hands-on from the master. The experience was awesome!

When I returned to California, the exercise strategies I learned helped me crush it in the gym. I had learned great new supplementation strategies to enhance fat loss, but the information that shocked me the most was the discussion we had about the one common thing that holds people back from getting results and performing at their highest levels.

The surprising roadblock? Sleep!

When I was younger, I had always viewed sleep as a sign of weakness. I truly believed you had to cheat sleep to achieve success. When he shared the nugget of information about its importance, I was utterly blown away. The man I admired so much totally shattered my beliefs about what it takes to become successful.

Why does this matter?

Cheating sleep is accompanied by serious health risks and has a major dampening effect on your overall performance. Studies show that a lack of sleep can cause us to gain weight and increase the risks of cardiovascular disease, high blood pressure, diabetes, and even mental disorders. Just to add an extra point to show how damaging lack of sleep is, cancer has actually been shown to grow two to three times faster in lab animals experiencing sleep dysfunction.

Research shows that our brains work much better with more sleep, allowing us to perform better on the field, in the office, and at home with those you love the most. Think about it. How much better do you function when you've had a good night's sleep rather than not enough?

Even so, there are many people who believe the need for sleep is a sign of weakness and laziness and a waste of time that robs our wallets. George Burns said it best: "Don't stay in bed unless you can make money in bed."

Even worse, there are those who think you must deprive yourself of sleep if you truly want to be successful. A survey presented in William C. Dement's book *The Promise of Sleep* shows that 80 percent of Americans actually believe you cannot be a success at work and at the same time get enough sleep. (As you will read later in this chapter, you *can* and *should* have both!)

Who developed *that* theory?

Believe it or not, it was the great overachiever himself, Thomas Edison, who was at the forefront of convincing us that sleep was for the weak. He prided himself on only sleeping 4 to 5 hours a night. For many, functioning on a lack of sleep, putting in long hours, and getting lots done has been a badge of honor, something to brag about.

I will admit there was a time in my life when I too believed that a lack of sleep was an essential requirement for success. I truly subscribed to the theory that if I wanted to get ahead in life, I had to outwork everyone else. That meant cheating sleep, burning the candle at both ends, and doing whatever it took to get the most hours out of each day. I still hear the motivational mantra I fell for at a young age,

"You can sleep when you're dead," or as Benjamin Franklin once put it, "There will be sleeping enough in the grave."

I've got some good news for you. By the end of this chapter, you, like many of my clients who have successfully done the Stark Naked 21-Day Metabolic Reset, will discover that getting 7 to 9 hours of sleep a night is one of the most important and vital components in

---

Marisol, schoolteacher, mother of two
California
Age forty-three

▶ *Marisol is an incredibly passionate teacher and mother of two great children. She loves the challenge and creativity required to keep her students focused, so she can guide and develop them, but her severe insomnia eventually caught up with her.*

When we first met, she struggled with how impatient and grumpy she had become with the students in her class and her own children. She was no longer the happy, creative, compassionate woman she once saw herself as. Marisol was tired of the belly fat she had accumulated and, worst of all, was literally tired of being tired all the time.

Her pattern was to grind and push through in spite of her fatigued state at all cost. In her mind, she had no option. She had to keep working. Eventually, that approach catches up with someone. She ended up crashing. She was getting sick often or finding herself unable to get out of bed for an entire weekend. This would happen multiple times every year.

When Marisol first came to me, her initial request, like that of so many others, was "Brad, I need an exercise plan to get rid of my belly. My current program is not working."

I knew Marisol would be disappointed when I told her exercise wasn't the answer she was looking for. She reluctantly agreed to

try the Stark Naked 21-Day Metabolic Reset, thinking I was off my rocker. It went against everything she, as an educator, thought she knew about fitness. Still, I convinced her we needed to deal with her fatigue first by helping her sleep again, if she truly wanted her old body back.

Within 3 days of starting the Reset, Marisol slept a full 7 hours without waking once during the night. Then it happened again, followed by another night, and then another. Marisol's fatigue slowly started to subside as her sleep became consistent, and her mood quickly began to change. Her improved sleep was leading to a more optimistic outlook; she was beginning to feel like her old self again.

By the end of the 21-Day Reset Marisol had completely rejuvenated her energy and creativity and was once again happy! She was actually having fun in her classroom and at home. Even her principal noticed a difference, not only with Marisol but also with Marisol's students. They were excelling in the classroom, because Marisol's enthusiasm was rubbing off on them.

Oh, yeah, I almost forgot. Marisol also lost 6 pounds and 3½ inches off her waist in the 21 days. As an added bonus, the acne she had struggled with her whole life also cleared up. Although this isn't an anticipated side effect for everyone, it certainly was one for her.

Marisol's metabolism had been shutting down because her liver was totally overwhelmed. It was making her sluggish, keeping her up at night, causing the weight gain on her belly, ruining her mood, and having a negative impact on her skin. Simply following the plan and loving her liver for 21 days allowed her to sleep again and greatly helped to completely reset her metabolism. Six months later she has kept the weight and inches off, and her sleep has remained amazing. She has not had an episode of crashing or getting sick in over six months and plans to maintain her newfound lifestyle for years to come.

your long-term success at everything you do. Not only will you discover the benefits of the Reset by improving the quality of your sleep; you will also learn to embrace the value of sleep. Once you do, you'll make sleep a priority.

Great success is achieved by finding the things others are unwilling to do and then doing them! Believe me, sleep is a part of that formula.

I love supporting high achievers, like you and Marisol, in this world. The impact you have is so powerful; one simple change like Marisol's can send out a ripple effect, creating change so vast you will never understand the impact a simple 21-day choice can make on the future of this world. There are enough tired, grumpy, irritable people in this world bringing it down. We need more people like you to make the change Marisol made and exude happiness, kindness, and passion for life.

Americans' Ongoing Struggle with Sleep

The CDC, in the April 27, 2012, issue of the *Morbidity and Mortality Weekly Report*, reported that 30 percent of all Americans are sleep deprived and are only getting 6 or less hours of sleep each night. They also found those who work more than 40 hours a week were dramatically more likely to be sleep deprived than those who worked 40 hours or less per week. According to some estimates, 90 percent of people with insomnia—a sleep disorder characterized by trouble falling and staying asleep—also have another health condition.

More than sixty million Americans struggle with getting enough sleep. If you're sleep deprived, meaning that you sleep 6 hours a night or less, you literally function as if you're under the influence of alcohol. This means that three out of every ten people around you right now are functioning as though they've been drinking. Now, there's a sobering thought!

I always tell my clients that the quickest way to keep themselves from being mediocre is to find a way to get 7 to 9 hours of deep rejuvenating sleep every night. When I share this information with my clients, most of them think that I'm nuts. In their mind, that's a third of their day. They can't give that precious time up for something as "wasteful" as sleep. But if they did, they, like you, would quickly discover that sleep is the greatest source of insane success and happiness.

Say what? The truth is, most people are struggling with issues that are preventing them from sleeping: stress, insomnia, disrupted sleep, or too many distractions in the bedroom, such as phones and other electronic devices that are not shut down at night. Whether you're aware of it or not, the sound of those devices dinging all night long actually interrupts your sleep. Your best bet is to shut those iPads and smartphones down for a good night's sleep.

Although the Stark Naked 21-Day Metabolic Reset can help resolve some of those physical issues, to reap the most benefits in the long run, once you feel better, you must commit to maintaining your sleep, or you will end up right back where you started—feeling horrible and run down in no time.

If I could promise you greater happiness and success in your life simply by challenging you to get more sleep, would you take that challenge?

Check this out. Science is now showing that *10* hours of sleep is ideal for extreme athletes. People who push their bodies to the limit actually need to give it more time to rest. Think about that for a second.

Look, I have studied the benefits of sleep on people from all walks of life. I have seen the impact it can have on energy, body composition, health, brain function, and happiness. It is extremely clear to me that people who make sleep a priority in their life have a tremendous advantage in all of those categories over those who choose to cheat sleep. It's the sine qua non for feeling, looking, and performing at your very best.

The Stark Naked 21-Day Metabolic Reset has been built on proven foundational strategies that will no doubt improve your sleep. Stress is the number one reason we fall victim to sleep disturbances, and the Reset is designed to attack that stress. Poor sleep is also a trigger for stress; therefore, once we reduce your stress, you will need strategies to protect your sleep long-term, so you don't end up back in the Metabolic Breakdown Cycle. At the end of this chapter, I will give you strategies to enhance and protect your precious sleep that I want you to start practicing now, so by the time you have completed your Reset, your sleep strategies will be dialed in.

I am such a great believer in the need for quality sleep that I have

---

Kendra, stay-at-home mom
Saskatchewan, Canada
Age thirty-three

▶ *Kendra is a stay-at-home mom of three. Before starting the Stark Naked 21-Day Metabolic Reset, she struggled with her weight after the birth of her last child and was frustrated by her lack of energy from sleep struggles. This combination made it difficult for her to survive her long days, let alone thrive during them.*

In the mornings, everyone knew to give mommy her space until she had her morning cup of coffee and some time to "wake up." Though she tried multiple diets and even attempted Cross-Fit to lose weight, she always seemed to find herself without the success she was looking for. Kendra got leaner and stronger, but the scale never changed. What Kendra really wanted was to see some weight drop on the scale.

The diets she tried were too restrictive for her. Within weeks she gave up on them. She was looking for a lifestyle change that would allow her to lose some weight, but one that would also increase her energy and provide options that didn't make it feel so

researched and developed strategies to not only help you fall sleep easier, but also improve the duration of your sleep. No more lying in bed waiting to fall asleep, or worse—no more nights of waking up between 1:00 and 3:00 A.M. and finding yourself unable to fall back asleep.

My wife, Maria, recently went back to work following her maternity leave after giving birth to our third child. During her first week back, our older children were on a week's vacation from school, and I got to stay home and watch them. As the week approached, my wife worried if I would be able to handle the responsibility. At the time, I couldn't understand why.

restrictive. As a busy mom, Kendra also struggled with sleep. Not only did she have trouble falling asleep, she also awoke during the night with a racing mind, which kept her up for hours.

Deep down, I knew if she was going to have any long-term success with losing weight, Kendra needed to improve the quality of her sleep. Within a week of starting the Stark Naked 21-Day Metabolic Reset, Kendra began to experience such a deep sleep that she started sleeping through the night for the first time in years. As soon as that happened, it wasn't long before the weight began to fall off. She lost 14 pounds within the first 21 days, and it's still coming off.

Kendra's weight loss took a backseat to the lifestyle changes she experienced from completing the Reset. Instead of being lethargic and grumpy in the morning, she was now energetic and happy. Her energy throughout the day went through the roof, allowing her to more effectively remain patient with her kids and provide a more engaged playful environment. She is now resilient to stress and in control of her world and the world she provides her children.

Four hours into day one I was exhausted! The energy required to keep up with our kids while caring for our new baby's needs was unbelievable. I was shocked by how tired I was at the end of the day—not to mention how grumpy I was! By late afternoon, the baby was crying, the older kids were complaining they were bored, and all I could wish was "Calgon, take me away!"

I was so relieved to have survived that week without any catastrophes, but even more so to go back to work. That was one of the most stressful, demanding, exhausting weeks I've had in a long time. Knowing how demanding being a stay-at-home parent is helped me understand my client Kendra's needs when she reached out to me desperate for answers to help her survive and thrive in the high-stress, demanding environment at home with young children.

The Risks of Sleep Deprivation

Don't sleep—at your own risk. But what happens when your lack of sleep puts others at risk?

Sleep deprivation has caused some of the greatest historic tragedies of the century. Not sure of what I am talking about? Ever hear of the Exxon Valdez oil spill, the space shuttle *Challenger* explosion, Chernobyl, Three Mile Island? All of these involved human error due to sleep deprivation.

If that seems too big to grasp, then look at it like this. Studies show that sleep loss and poor-quality sleep also lead to accidents and injuries on the job. In one study, workers who complained about excessive daytime sleepiness had significantly more work accidents, particularly repeated work accidents. They also had more sick days per accident. That might not mean that much to the average employee, but to a business owner that adds up to a lot of dollars.

Lack of sleep can slow reaction time as much as drinking does, and both impair driving. Fatigue from lack of sleep is estimated to cause around 100,000 auto crashes and more than 1,550 crash-related deaths a year. In the "Sleep in America" poll, taken by the National Sleep Foundation, 37 percent of Americans (103 million people) admitted to falling asleep while driving in 2011.

I remember a near disaster that almost ruined my life in my mid-twenties. I was training clients starting at 5:00 A.M. usually until 6:00 P.M. From there I would head to my second job of bartending special events. I could be out as late as 2:00 A.M. on some nights. Although I was making great money, I was severely sleep deprived. Even so, I was very proud of my intense work ethic, which was, in my mind, helping me climb that "ladder of success."

I had finished an event one Saturday around 8:00 P.M. I had been bartending at the beach and was driving back to my company's head-quarters to return the bar equipment and remaining alcohol. I was exhausted from being out in the sun all day and having a ridiculously long week. I had the AC cranked up in the car and the windows rolled down. I was trying anything I could think of to keep myself awake at the wheel. Unfortunately, it wasn't working very well. My eyes were heavy and I could feel my head bobbing around as I began drifting in and out of consciousness. I came up to an intersection and didn't notice the couple in the crosswalk with their toddler and a baby in a stroller. Thankfully, they saw me and quickly realized I wasn't slowing down for the red light. They backpedaled toward the sidewalk as I blew through the light. I came to as I just missed crushing the baby stroller.

Looking into those parents' eyes as I whizzed by, seeing their fear and their anger, and then experiencing my own guilt for what I had almost done is something I will never forget. My heart was racing, and I was panic-stricken by what had nearly transpired. I had no problem staying awake for the remainder of my drive, but I quickly gave up my bartending job. I couldn't handle the long hours and lack of sleep. It was taking a toll on my body, and I almost paid a price that was too high to ignore.

To this day I am no longer willing to drive if I am even the slightest bit tired or fatigued.

Cheating Sleep Is Making You Fat

The reality is, when you don't sleep, you are totally disrupting your hormones. These fluctuations range from an elevated appetite to collapsing sex hormones. It only takes one night of not sleeping enough to trigger a negative response. For example, one night of sleeping only 4 hours will cause your hunger to spike and your blood-sugar and insulin levels to take on the characteristics of insulin resistance (the prediabetic stage). In this condition you can't process carbohydrates properly, yet you crave carbohydrate-rich foods the following day, like breads, pastries, and candy, which end up being stored as fat instead of muscle.

The University of Chicago reported research showing that morning testosterone levels can drop by as much as 60 percent for those sleeping 4 hours instead 8. Combining these responses with the elevation in cortisol we talked about earlier and you have the perfect recipe for fat storage. You've been bombarded with the message that you simply need to exercise more and eat less to rev up your metabolism, but in reality the first place you must start is with your sleep.

Recent research has focused on the link between sleep and the peptides that regulate appetite. Ghrelin stimulates hunger, and leptin signals satiety to the brain and suppresses appetite. Shortened sleep time is associated with decreases in leptin and elevations in ghrelin, leading many people to be hungrier than usual the following day. To make matters even worse, sleep debt has a negative effect on the brain as well, because it impairs the frontal lobe, which is responsible for judgment, and stimulates the part of the brain that controls motivation and desire.

When you impair judgment while stimulating desire and increasing hunger, you create the perfect storm for creating and satisfying your cravings for your favorite high-fat, high-carbohydrate foods, like ice cream. That's why those people in the earlier study who only slept 4 hours a night were 73 percent more likely to be obese than those who slept 7 to 9 hours a night.

Lack of Sleep and Its Impact on Mojo

"Not tonight, dear. I'm too tired."

Are those words that have become all too familiar in your bedroom?

Sleep specialists say that sleep-deprived men and women report lower libidos and less interest in sex.

Depleted energy, sleepiness, and increased tension may be largely to blame. We already know that increased cortisol can impact just about everything! However, a recent study funded by the National Heart, Lung, and Blood Institute found testosterone levels dropped significantly in men who don't get enough sleep—the levels were the equivalent of those for men 10 to 15 years older. That explains the lack of sex drive, but lower testosterone can bring about other negative side effects, especially for younger men, including reduced libido and poor reproduction. But they may even find themselves unable to build enough strength through muscle mass and bone density, leading to lower energy levels, poor concentration, and chronic fatigue. Low testosterone levels are also linked to metabolic syndrome—a cluster of metabolic risk factors that increase the chances of developing heart disease, stroke, and type 2 diabetes.

Long-term sleep deprivation leaves major, long-lasting effects on hormone levels. Scientists from the University of Chicago found men who get less than 5 hours of sleep a night for a week or longer suffer from dramatically lower levels of testosterone than those who get a good night's rest. Their study, published in the *Journal of the Ameri-*

can Medical Association, found that the levels of the hormone are reduced dramatically to levels more similar to those 15 years older.

Lack of Sleep and Depression

Over the years, I've noticed that a lot of the high achievers I've come into contact with deal with bouts of depression. For them, it seems to come out of the blue. They feel blindsided. Interestingly, many of those people are also severely sleep deprived. In fact, most would be clinically labeled as insomniacs.

Trouble sleeping can be one of the first symptoms of depression. Research has shown there is a lot of correlation between insomnia and depression. One large study of ten thousand people, published in the journal *Sleep,* found that people suffering from insomnia were *5 times* more likely to develop depression! One of the best ways to improve mood and maintain a positive, happy outlook on life is to get enough sleep. Look, I know it's a lot easier said than done for those who can't sleep. But understand, if you're not sleeping, something is wrong.

What Professional Athletes
Know About Sleep That You Should Too

A number of great athletes today share one common focus—sleep! I've read that LeBron James sleeps 12 hours a night. Roger Federer sleeps 11 to 12 hours a night. Usain Bolt, 8 to 10 hours. Venus Williams, 8 to 10 hours. Michelle Wie, 10 to 12 hours.

Highly trained athletes tend to be way ahead of the curve when it comes to taking care of their bodies. The rest of us who actually care about ourselves follow suit a few years down the road. Core training and functional exercise were once thought of as exclusive training techniques for the elite athletes of the world, but now most every trainer I know uses these methods with their clients. Current trends such as heart-rate variability monitoring for readiness levels and something called fatigue science—also known as the study of the impact of sleep deprivation—are at the forefront of cutting-edge training today. Fatigue science has become so hot that the San Francisco Giants used a well-known sleep expert, Dr. Chris Winter, to help give them a competitive advantage in winning the 2014 World Series.

In November 2012, the *Wall Street Journal* article "Sleeping Your Way to the Top" shared strategies from three NFL teams focusing on sleep to help improve field performance. Two of the three teams featured, the San Francisco 49ers and the Baltimore Ravens, eventually met in the Super Bowl a couple of months later. Some might write that fact off as a coincidence, but I wouldn't dare. These teams put a massive emphasis on the body's need for sleep, following scientific research showing that sleep enhances athleticism and gives a huge competitive advantage.

The Stanford University Center for Sleep Sciences and Medicine has been extensively studying the effects of extended sleep on athletic performance. In one study the researchers asked athletes from a variety of sports to focus on extending their sleep to at least 10 hours a night. The results were staggering.

Swimmers experienced increases in speed, improved reaction time off the blocks, faster turns, and increased kick strokes. Tennis players improved sprinting speed and serving accuracy. Football players experienced an improvement in their 40-yard-dash time by an average of $\frac{1}{10}$ of a second. I know a lot of NFL hopefuls who have paid thousands of dollars to shave $\frac{1}{10}$ of a second off their 40-yard dash. That $\frac{1}{10}$ of a second can be worth millions of dollars. Basketball players experienced huge increases in shooting accuracy.

There is also extensive research showing that when athletes get more rest, there is a major reduction in the risk of injuries. Naturally, this is optimal for those who rely on their body to function in peak condition day in and day out.

One study of teenage athletes found that those who slept at least 8 hours a night had a 68 percent reduction in injury risk compared to those who slept less than 8 hours a night. Talk to most teenagers today. They get nowhere near 8 hours of sleep, with their demanding schedules that include practice time, schoolwork, and other activities. It's no wonder injuries have steadily been on the rise for our high-school athletes.

Here's the bottom line. If you're an athlete looking for a competitive advantage that also reduces your risk of injury, you must put a major focus on getting more sleep. Start targeting 10 hours of sleep every night. It will absolutely help take your game to the next level. I guarantee it! There is no diet or training program that will provide the same reward in performance as optimal sleep.

The Advantages of Sleep Outside of Sports

Athletes are not the only ones who can enjoy the advantage of improved performance from sleep. We can all benefit from getting a good night's sleep. That's why getting 7 to 9 hours of sleep each night is one of the key components in the Stark Naked 21-Day Metabolic Reset. To further validate this connection between enhanced performance and quantity of sleep, let's take a moment and analyze what prevents most people from getting enough sleep in the first place.

Dr. K. Anders Ericsson did a famous study that declared it takes 10,000 hours of deliberate practice to become great at something. Most people who know about this study use it to validate their depriving themselves of sleep in order to get more done trying to reach greatness in the first place. Interestingly, there was one additional factor in that same study regarding performance that few people talk about. The highest performers in Dr. Ericsson's study also slept an average of 8 hours and 36 minutes a night.

Yes, they got over 8 hours of sleep a night. When was the last time you got 8½ hours of quality sleep? Sleep is critical to whatever you're chasing in life.

When you get the optimum amount of sleep, not only will your body operate better physically; your mind will function better too. Your thoughts will be clearer and more cohesive. You will be more alert and aware of everything in your surroundings. Dr. William C. Dement, in *The Promise of Sleep*, explores how sleep affects overall performance by looking at things like the ability to receive information, the ability to act on information, and the individual attention span. To support his findings, he turned to research from fatigue expert David Dinges, at the University of Pennsylvania, who found that when people were forced to sleep 4 hours a night for two weeks, their performance in these categories was severely impaired, especially toward the end of the 14 days. Basically, sleep loss made people stupid.

I don't know about you, but I completely know how that feels. As a new dad, I know there are plenty of mornings I wonder if I should even be driving a car! As soon as I can catch a nap, my mind and thoughts realign.

The performance advantages from enhanced sleep seen on the sporting fields were due to more than just better physical recovery. Physical repair and muscular recovery are definitely enhanced by more sleep, but two other key benefits of greater sleep are vital for high achievers in any arena: better cognitive function and better stress control. Dr. Michael Breus, known as the "Sleep Doctor," also feels that cognitive benefits play a huge role in enhancing the athletes' performance. Everyone can benefit from a brain that makes quicker, more accurate decisions. It doesn't take much to slow things down— just one night of sleep deprivation can decrease response time.

It should also come as no surprise that not getting enough sleep triggers the stress response in our bodies. Research on nonathlete populations found that those who are sleep deprived have much higher levels of cortisol in their blood the following day, and it takes up to six times longer to return to normal than for those in the control groups. Now that you know how damaging cortisol can be when its level is chronically elevated, simply getting more z's can build resiliency against cortisol. Simply stated, those who get more sleep are basically calmer and happier people, two great characteristics for better performance in any environment!

Most people are proud to show off their sleep deprivation as a badge of honor around the water cooler, but what they don't realize is how badly their lack of sleep is robbing them of their energy and mental ability to work at their highest level. Sure, they might be at the office, working long hours day in and day out, but they are likely not functioning in the most productive manner. If they are actually mentally checked out, completing mediocre work and getting a fraction of the work done in twice the amount of time, what's the point of punching the clock? If you want to stand out at work, increase your sleep. Within a matter of days of sleeping more these are the benefits you can expect to experience:

Better decision making

Better attention span

Better memory

Increased energy and reduced afternoon energy slump

Improved mood and therefore better working relationships

Increased motivation

Less risk of on-the-job injury

Less anxiety

Better ability to handle stress

More creativity

Better problem-solving skills

The Foundation for Great Sleep

Now that you understand the importance of sleep, I want to help you set up the best environment for it. There are two strategies I have learned over the years that are the foundation for a great night's sleep. These strategies are going to take a little extra effort on your part, but they are worth it.

The Stark Naked 21-Day Metabolic Reset will improve your internal environment and provide you with better-quality sleep, but if your external environment isn't in sync with these new changes, it will prevent you from having an optimum experience. To allow for a great night's sleep you must first set your room up. Once you've done that, you'll warm up for sleep each night just as you should warm up before you exercise.

The Bat Cave

I first learned about the "bat-cave theory" in 2007 at a Biosignature Seminar with Charles Poliquin. The bat-cave theory is simply the idea of making your bedroom resemble a bat cave. Dark and cold is the ultimate answer for great sleep. The darker the room, the more melatonin you produce, which allows for a more regenerative sleep. The temperature of your room should generally be cool.

On any given day, your body temperature naturally rises and drops. In the evening, your temperature naturally drops as your body gets tired, and at night it actually reaches its lowest point around 5:00 A.M.

We've all experienced how hard it is to sleep in a hot room. For most people, it's a frustrating night of tossing and turning combined with very little sleep. For optimal sleep, the ideal temperature of your bedroom should be between 65 and 72 degrees. The colder, the better, as your body needs to cool down to induce sleep. If your bedroom is too hot, it can cause insomnia, because your body cannot naturally cool down. As an added bonus, there is some scientific support that shows sleeping in a cooler room can even help you burn fat while you're asleep.

It's also important to keep your head cool. Research shows that the brain prefers being cooler to enhance sleep. A hot pillow can cause sleep issues. In a study done by the University of Pittsburgh School of Medicine, insomniacs who wore a cooling cap had an easier time falling asleep and stayed asleep dramatically longer.

Strategies to Create Your Bat Cave

- Put up blackout shades to create complete darkness. I want your room so dark you can't even see your hand in front of your face. It's a little eerie at first, but the payoff in better sleep is so worthwhile. Prices for blackout shades range from $30 to $200-plus, depending on quality and the size and number of windows.
- Set your thermostat at 65–72 degrees. This is the ideal temperature for sleep.
- Sleep with minimal clothing on to help keep body temperature down.
- Remove anything that is plugged in from your room. The bat cave is literally for the two best things in life: sleep and sex.

Warm Up for Better Sleep

The bat cave is an incredible setting for deeper and better sleep, but if you don't apply specific strategies before getting into bed, you can still end up staring into the darkness unable to check out. You have got to unplug from your overly stimulating world. Your brain and nervous system need a chance to calm down and allow the process of sleep induction to kick in. To warm up for better sleep, apply the following strategies:

- One hour before bed, unplug from the world by turning off the TV, computer, iPad, smartphone, and so on. The blue light that is emitted from these devices tells the brain it's light outside and therefore it's time to wake up—not sleep. Unplug from these and spend some time reading by yourself, read with your kids, talk with your significant other, take a warm bath, or meditate— anything that will reconnect you with yourself and those you love the most.

- Create and keep a Gratitude Journal. One of the most powerful tools I have found to date is writing in a gratitude journal each night before bed. Simply writing down three to five things you're thankful for each night before turning out the light is huge for enhancing sleep—and your life.

Sometimes duty calls, and we have to get on the computer in the evening. Choose screens that don't interfere with your sleep if you can and keep use to a minimum. To prevent insomnia from blue-light exposure, I have Flux installed on my Mac. In the evening it emits a light that is more red than blue to help keep my brain calm, so I can still easily fall asleep. I use the computer sparingly during this time, as I like to separate from my work as much as possible each night, so my sleep is not hampered.

I know, we are so used to being connected to the rest of the world through our tech devices these days that unplugging may be difficult. But give it a try for the next 21 days and see how it impacts your sleep.

Strategies for Challenging Sleep Issues

If you've applied the above strategies and sleep is still an issue, here are some advanced strategies for improving sleep. At Stark we find that clients usually fall into one of two camps: either they struggle falling asleep or they crash easily but can't stay asleep.

Trouble Falling Asleep

If you have a hard time falling asleep and the foundation strategies of the bat cave and warming up for bed have not worked, you're dealing with a source of unwanted stress before bed that needs to be calmed down. Try the following solutions.

Drink tart cherry juice. Two separate research studies have shown that people who drank two small glasses of tart cherry juice a day significantly improved the quality of sleep and increased its duration. Tart cherry juice works because it naturally raises your melatonin levels, which have been shown to have an influence on quality of sleep by regulating your sleeping-waking cycle. These studies also showed that people who consumed the tart cherry juice in the morning and before bed actually took fewer naps during the day, meaning they had more energy.

Do a deep-breathing meditation. Simple breathing strategies can really help calm down unwanted stress. Try using a relaxed deep-breathing technique: sit or lie in a very comfortable position, keep your eyes closed, and breathe in through your nose for 4 seconds and out through your mouth for 4 seconds. Focus on deep abdominal breaths; with each breath, you should feel your belly rise as you breathe in and fall as you breathe out.

Trouble Staying Asleep

If you fall asleep on the couch or are out cold within 5 minutes of lying down, you are showing the classic signs of sleep deprivation, but many of you struggle with sleeping through the whole night. It's become obvious people usually wake in one of two windows of time. Most high performers either wake between 1:00 and 3:00 or between 3:00 and 5:00 A.M. Let's explore some solutions you can try to better improve your sleep during these periods.

Waking Between 1:00 and 3:00 A.M.

I would guess somewhere between 80 and 90 percent of all high achievers we work with struggle with waking between 1:00 and 3:00 A.M. when they first come in. Usually this is due to dips in blood sugar at night, forcing the adrenals to pump cortisol to stabilize blood sugar, which wakes you up. Eating a snack before bed to make sure blood sugar stays stable is built into the Stark Naked 21-Day Metabolic Reset and usually solves this problem. If you are skipping this snack because you still believe eating before bed will make you fat and you are waking between 1:00 and 3:00 A.M., do yourself a favor and have the snack—problem solved. If you're eating the snack, then here is another solution you can try.

Chinese medicine shows us that people who wake between 1:00 and 3:00 A.M. are having issues with their liver meridian. Have you ever noticed that when you drink a little too much alcohol, you fall asleep quickly but end up waking sometime between 1:00 and 3:00 A.M. and then struggle with sleeping the remainder of the night?

Dr. Dayne Grove, the Stark staff doctor of naturopathy and Chinese medicine, chooses to put our clients on a "liver tonic" as his first option for treating those waking during this window. Their immediate improvement in sleep is incredible. To battle this naturally, I have purposely built green tea into the daily outline in the afternoon. Green tea has a lot of liver-support qualities and also has an amino acid called L-theanine, which helps calm stress. If you are waking between 1:00 and 3:00, it's really important to drink the afternoon green tea during your reset.

Waking Between 3:00 and 5:00 A.M.

Waking between 3:00 and 5:00 A.M. is linked to the lungs in Chinese medicine, and excessive oxidative stress tends to be the cause. The answer here is to add more antioxidants into your daily diet. A good first solution will be making sure you use dark-skinned fruit as your nighttime snack before going to bed during the Reset, which you will read more about in Chapter 11. Dark-skinned fruits have more antioxidants. These include fruits like plums, berries, and cherries. The tart cherry juice discussed earlier is great for solving this sleep issue as well.

Applying these strategies can only improve the quality and duration of your sleep, supplying you with more energy, better focus, an uplifted mood, more sex drive, and a better body to enjoy sex with. Remember, sleep is the most critical component to your long-term success.

> Getting 7 to 9 hours of sleep a night is essential to your long-term success in everything you do. The Reset will improve your quality of sleep, resulting in better body and brain function.

Chris, CEO, Pure Game, age forty-seven
Tony, founder, Pure Game, age forty-seven
California

▶ *Chris and Tony run a nonprofit organization called Pure Game, which focuses on developing character in at-risk children through experiential learning. They use the game of soccer to help children break free from their current situations and negative mindsets. Imagine the energy needed to run around on the soccer fields all day teaching and mentoring at-risk children.*

When we first met, Chris and Tony both struggled with sleep, leaving them dragging most of the time. They needed coffee and caffeinated teas to help push them through their days. Their hearts were in the right place, but their bodies wanted to be home in bed—catching up on their lost sleep.

When the two men started the Stark Naked 21-Day Metabolic Reset, I purposely had them start on a Friday. I knew they would struggle for the first few days once I removed their false energy source—caffeine—and I didn't want that to affect the kids they worked with.

As expected, they were both miserable for the first 3 days. They slept a lot due to their true low-energy state. Tony's sleep quickly became regulated, though. He began sleeping through the night in no time. I am always amazed at how much better most people sleep once I remove the stimulant caffeine. In fact, he was hitting such deep levels of sleep that he would sleep right through the crying of one of his own children during the night. His wife would have to wake him to go get their child!

Chris took a little longer to regulate, but by day 10 of the Reset, his sleep had settled in nicely too. Up until then, Chris had been routinely getting sinus infections that would keep him up at night. Ever since starting this program, however, his sinus infections have been greatly controlled, allowing him to sleep better and longer.

Together, their energy on the field is incredible! Their ability to lead their organization has dramatically improved, and their impact is growing at an incredible rate. The power of sleep is truly amazing! Tony and Chris are changing the future of our society and now they have the energy and stamina to impact and change the trajectory of lives for even more vulnerable children.

9

Exercise

Why *Less* Is More!

W HEN YOU SEE THE WORD "exercise," what do you associate with it? The most common response I get from clients is "punishment." These responders are divided into two camps:

Camp 1: Exercise is a bad punishment, so I am going to completely avoid it.

Camp 2: Exercise is a good punishment. The more I can suffer through, the better it is going to be for me.

Which camp would you pitch your tent in?

But guess what? The people in both camps are robbing themselves of their best possible lives. Why?

Both versions of "exercise is punishment" lead to excessive amounts of unneeded stress on the body, stealing your energy and happiness, increasing your likelihood of getting sick, accelerating your aging process, blocking your creativity, and destroying your desire to roll in the hay.

Those of you who currently live in the "exercise is bad punishment" camp probably bought this book believing it would be another prescription touting the notion, "Exercise is a must for success." You'd be partially right. Keep reading, because I think you're going to like what I have to say about exercise. By the end of this chapter you will see that more is not necessarily better, and as a result you may just change your stance.

Exercise Is Bad Punishment and Must Be Avoided

Exercise is a gift, a reward that a healthy body craves. It's my belief that if your body doesn't want to move, then your metabolism is most likely broken and needs to be resuscitated—or, as I like to say, reset.

When I first met my client Brandon, he was overweight and felt miserable. Brandon, forty-two, is the owner of a commodities-trading company. He weighed 320 pounds and slept somewhere between 2 and 4 hours a night. He had dark circles under his eyes, looked perpetually exhausted, and walked around radiating how miserable he felt to the world. The guy was suffering and was eager to make some vast changes. He was desperate to lose the excess weight he had somehow accumulated over the past few years. I will never forget the first words he said to me when we met.

"Brad, I haven't exercised in fifteen years, and I hate it. I know you're going to tell me I need to exercise. If that's your resolution to getting me fit again, this meeting is over. I will not exercise!"

Yeah, I could see I had my work cut out for me, but I knew Brandon wasn't a lost cause. In fact, he was my ideal client.

With a big smile on my face, I replied, "No problem, buddy. For the first 21 days as my client you're not allowed to exercise, so don't even ask."

The look on his face was classic. I think his jaw hit the table, because no trainer had ever said that to him before. Like most people, Brandon had been misled into believing that exercise was the ultimate answer to getting healthy, and unless he was willing to hop on that train, he would never get results.

By now of course, you know I had a different plan for Brandon. Within the first week of starting the Stark Naked 21-Day Metabolic Reset, Brandon was sleeping a solid and valuable 8 hours a night—every night. The weight started to peel off rather quickly and without a lot of effort or pain.

Around 15 days in, my phone rang. It was Brandon calling to tell me he had so much energy that he was actually ready to start working out. I reminded him that our agreement was no exercise for the first 21 days.

"Call me on day 22," I said.

I knew what I was doing. You see, with a guy like Brandon, exercise was something I needed him to want. I couldn't force it. Not now, not ever. The longer I made him wait for it, the more he would want it. Sure, I have clients who exercise moderately during the 21-Day Reset period because they thrive on exercise, but these are high achievers who are cutting back—not starting a regime for the very first time.

When day 22 came, you can bet the first call I got that morning was from Brandon. He was begging me to exercise. In three weeks, he had dropped 17 pounds and 3 inches off his waist. He was now sleeping throughout the night, and his energy was off the charts. He was rested, energetic, and in a much better mood. His wife wanted to know what I had done with her old husband. He was a completely different man after just 21 days. Best of all, the man who once viewed exercise as the ultimate punishment was now eager and excited about it! His punishment had become his ultimate reward. Six months after starting his reset, Brandon has lost 70 pounds and continues to follow the program. One thing is for sure, he is *never* going back to his old unhealthy, sedentary lifestyle.

Once you make a shift in your thinking and see the value in taking care of yourself as a reward and not a punishment, you will start to unleash the true power of great health and fitness that lives inside each and every one of us. You will no longer despise the effort. You will embrace the process.

How do you make that shift? Simply follow this program and allow your metabolism to be reset. You've got to relax and conquer!

If you're like Brandon and see exercise as a form of punishment or as the last thing you want to do for yourself, then don't exercise for the next 21 days (as long as you're on the Reset plan). I promise, by day 22, like Brandon, you're going to crave movement!

I have yet to see anyone who hated the punishment of exercise complete the 21-Day Reset and not be ready and willing to exercise. It's not going to be you, is it?

Exercise Is a Good Punishment and Must Be Endured

Not long ago, I received an e-mail from another well-known professional CrossFit athlete, the New Zealander Ruth Anderson-Horrell, who was pursuing the title of "Fittest on Earth." Like Becca Voigt, Ruth, age thirty, competed in the CrossFit Games multiple times. In her e-mail she wrote that her stomach was severely bloated from water retention, her body fat was creeping up even though she was exercising like crazy, she was moody, her strength was dwindling, and overall her gas tank felt as if it was on empty all the time. Additionally, she was experiencing dizziness and nausea after certain types of short, high-intensity bursts of exercise. After investigating her daily routine more thoroughly, I quickly discovered her recovery methods were not appropriately offsetting her training volume, and her body was starting to give up. The stress from exercise was literally killing her body and making Ruth and everyone around her miserable.

After talking it over with Ruth and her CrossFit coach, Dusty, we decided the answer was to shut down training for a period of time, so we could reset her metabolism. Ruth agreed to follow the Stark Naked 21-Day Metabolic Reset to the letter along with focusing on getting 10 hours of sleep a night to really allow her body to replenish her diminished energy reserves.

The only exercise she was allowed to do for the first 7 days was recovery exercise. Together, we chose walking in nature for her.

Walking in nature? Really?

Yes! Believe it or not, it's such a powerful form of exercise to reduce stress and aid in accelerating recovery. Research done by the University of Michigan has confirmed that walking in nature does wonders for improving mental health and reducing perceived stress. Spending time in nature is also great for lowering blood pressure, heart rate, and stress load on the central nervous system. According to Yoshifumi Miyazaki, Japan's leading scholar on forest therapy, walking in the woods relieves stress and helps the immune system recover more efficiently. Miyazaki's research on walking in nature not only validated the previous benefits; he also found it created a general relaxation of the body, decreased the stress hormone cortisol, decreased fatigue, and increased psychological vigor. These were all things Ruth could benefit from in her overstressed and tired state, so it was a logical choice.

In the second week we allowed Ruth to add in 2 days of short higher-intensity strength-training workouts to make sure she was able to maintain her strength and not lose too much ground during her recovery phase.

At the end of the initial 21-Day Reset, Ruth was scheduled to compete in a CrossFit event. Her results were amazing. By dramatically reducing her training volume and focusing only on recovery for the

21 days prior to the event, she crushed the initial 3-kilometer run straight uphill, then back down, without any energy issues and completed 2 more days of competing in multiple fitness events without feeling fatigued or running out of energy. Her strength did not falter, as so many people expected it would because she had reduced her training volume. She had done no special training for this event. She had only rested and reset prior to competing.

Ruth's situation is a classic example of "fatigue masking fitness." Thankfully Charles Poliquin had made me aware of this phenomenon years ago by teaching me that *exercise is worthless if you aren't successfully recovering from it.* Ruth was like so many of you who believe more exercise is good punishment and are therefore overstressing your bodies, which is ultimately leading to severe fatigue and metabolic breakdown.

I don't want you to suffer from that anymore. Your metabolism needs a reset! It's time to take a 21-day break from your intense exercise.

As hard as it may be for you to cut back at first, try to remember Ruth's amazing results. She felt better, performed better, and received numerous compliments about how great she looked at the end of the 21 days.

Now, I think it is only fair to share that I originally didn't believe Charles's thinking on recovery. I thought more had to be better. I never focused on recovery. I took great pride in my extreme commitment to excessive exercise and my refusal to rest in between workout days, and yes, although I ended up with a body that looked great, I felt horrible. The *best* I ever looked in life was the *worst* I ever felt.

I guess you can say I've always been a glutton for punishment and used to have a tendency learn things the hard way. A lot of these exercise ideas that are considered great at quickly changing our weight, body fat, and muscle levels are also great ways to ruin our energy, happiness, and sex drive. When I finally realized the value of recovery, everything changed. It was a real "aha" moment for me. And I want it to be one for you too.

The Stark Naked Exercise Theory

The clients I have worked with over the years have led me to some interesting perspectives on health, fitness, and performance, especially for high achievers. The reality is that most of us after the age of thirty have basically lost the desire to look like a Spartan warrior or a Victoria's Secret model.

I said most. There are still a few of you out there, and you know who you are.

For the most part, by the time you've reached this stage in life, you've likely realized you've got a lot more important things to focus on than spending your day living in the gym obsessing over your abs.

Do you still want to look good in a swimsuit on your vacation? Heck, yeah! But do you want to spend 2 hours a day in the gym slaving away for it, making yourself miserable and starving yourself to get there? No way! You have more important things to do with your time. You have bigger responsibilities that require a lot more energy to take care of.

It took me a while, but in my early thirties I finally figured out that it takes a whole lot more than a hard, chiseled body to attract a quality woman. Now that I am a husband and father, my number one priority is to have the energy for quality time with those I love after putting in a long day at work, great stamina to have a long successful career, and insane health to give myself the best chance of waking up every morning on this side of the dirt for many years to come.

And if you are like my clients, this is what many of you truly crave too. The disconnect for people is that, when it comes to exercise, most of the information on fitness and nutrition isn't focused on these goals. It's focused on appearance. That's why you are probably exhausted, wiped out by stress, and yet still forcing yourself out of bed every morning to get to that spin class or run 3 miles before the sun comes up, thinking you are doing something great for your body. Sadly, most of you have been brainwashed into believing you must exercise hard to be successful. Worse, many of you believe the more *fit* people are, the *healthier* they are.

Well, like many other mistaken notions, I'm about to shatter that myth too.

The Stark Naked strategies on exercise shared in this chapter are the same tactics I ultimately used to restore my life and fitness and the exact protocols I recommend when restoring those for all of my clients. These exercise strategies will teach you how to use exercise to accompany your Stark Naked 21-day Metabolic Reset and enhance your energy, motivation, happiness, health, and sex drive.

Personal experience has changed my perspective on what our exercise needs really are when our lives become complicated with responsibilities and pursuits. I have more compassion and understanding than most trainers, because my life closely resembles the lives of many of you. I am so much more than a trainer these days. You see, my old life as a trainer was simple. I didn't have much responsibility outside of training my clients and focusing on exercise to look good. In my current life I have a family, am a partner in a business, travel the world for more than a hundred speaking engagements a year, and run multiple full-immersion destination retreats. My perspective on exercise needs has dramatically changed. Looks are still important, but without great energy I am worthless when it comes to keeping up with all of my responsibilities and pursuits. Unfortunately, I have learned that the hard way too!

Before I had children, I could never understand why people with young children looked so tired and worn-out all the time. My inner thought was "How hard can it really be to take care of little ones?"

At the time, it seemed pretty obvious to me. I thought these people simply didn't care how they looked.

That all changed the day I became a dad. *Wow!* I was shocked at how fast I got fat after our first baby.

Some mornings it took every last drop of energy in me just to peel my face off the pillow and go to work. The idea of working out myself was just too much! Instead, I used that time to steal a quick nap. My sleeping times were not up to me anymore. I could no longer be lazy and just lay on the couch all day on Sunday. I had dad duty.

Oh, yeah. I sing a much different tune these days. Now I have so much compassion for new parents, because they have no idea what lies ahead. Before I had kids, I thought the answer was easy. You just need to suck it up and add more time in the gym to ward off the accumulating fat, but in reality that's the worst call.

Another eye-opening experience for me came over the last few years and has led me to become an effective coach for busy working professionals. I always assumed sitting at a desk all day was easy and could never understand why travel took such a toll on people's bodies. I figured it was simply an issue of laziness and all these people needed was more exercise and better direction in food choices. I remember when I received my first fitness tracker as a gift. It was the original Nike Fuelband. At the time, I thought the 10,000-steps-a-day rule was a joke. In my mind, I'd reached 10,000 steps by 10:00 A.M. every day as a trainer. It seemed to be setting the bar too low.

Fast-forward a few years. Today I spend around 6 to 8 hours a day seated in front of my computer screen working. By 7:00 P.M. most days I have only accumulated 3,000 steps for the day. Life can change pretty fast when you find yourself busy doing things other than being a personal trainer. Looks like I need to go for a walk before bed.

I value the feedback of my fitness tracker now, because I am shocked at how little I move in my new life. In fact, it serves as a nice reminder to get up and move. I am equally surprised at how tired and stiff my body gets just sitting all day. Some days, no, make that most days, the last thing I want to do after being glued to my computer screen for hours is exercise. It takes me a lot longer to warm up than it used to, so I can get a good workout in.

But I do it. Why? Because I know it's good for my mind, body, and spirit, which makes it good for my total health.

The secret to long-term change and enjoying a great high-performance lifestyle with a great body is to switch from the belief that looking a certain way or weighing a certain number is better than first feeling great! Once you start feeling great, you will quickly begin to look and perform great in *all* areas of your life. When you focus on how you feel, specifically your greatest asset, energy, you are bringing your metabolism back online and onto your side.

When you punish your body and focus only on how you look, you abuse your metabolism and are therefore forced to fight it. That is why you feel so bad!

The Stark Naked 21-Day Metabolic Reset Exercise System

Before I present the Stark Naked exercise system, let me be very clear: as a trainer I do not develop weak, slow, skinny people. The people I work with are not on a twelve-week transformation challenge just to look great in the mirror. Their lives, like yours, are very complex. Their training and performance requirements are complex and require year-round focus, which creates amazing stamina, enabling them to perform for years to come. The system I am about to share with you is highly tested and proven. It is currently being used by professional athletes, SWAT team members, CEOs, sports agents, CrossFit athletes, famous speakers, authors, Hollywood stuntmen, pastors, busy moms, high-performing businessmen and businesswomen, my wife after our third baby, and myself—just to name a few high achievers.

I don't build weak people. I build long-term, resilient high achievers. With this strategy you will get the most out of your body for the rest of your life.

Remember, intense exercise, which I love, like high-intensity interval training, lifting weights, spin class, and boot camps, are applying stress to your body. Extended overexposure to stress is at the core of your broken metabolism. I've said before and I'll say it again: *you cannot beat a stress-based problem by throwing more stress at it.*

You also cannot develop a resiliency to stress if you have not recovered from the damage of your past stress. Like any professional athlete, you need an off-season!

When you're trying to mend a broken metabolism, you have to remove as much unneeded stress as possible from the body, especially while you are resetting it. That's why we reduce intense exercise during the 21 days of your reset.

It's only three weeks! Your body will not fall apart! Remember, Ruth's body actually looked better and had better energy and strength in competition after she dramatically reduced her exercise volume for three weeks. Think of this as your personal off-season.

Here are a few of my favorite ways to focus on recovery:

Take a relaxing walk in nature. (Personally, I love the beach!)

Take a 10- to 30-minute catnap daily. (NASA uses this strategy with its astronauts, because it helps their brains work better.)

Get a massage, but avoid deep-tissue work, as pain creates stress. Get one of those relaxing Swedish rubdowns that makes you fall asleep and drool.

Do daily stretching and mobility work.

Practice meditation.

Get an acupuncture treatment.

Do cardiac output exercise, which is aerobic exercise that calms the body down. Try keeping your heart rate around 130 beats per minute (bpm; beats per minute can be tracked on a heart-rate monitor). Joel Jamieson taught me the value of this three years ago and it was life-changing for my fitness.

Here are my current daily, weekly, monthly recovery strategies:

Daily	Weekly	Monthly
Evening walks outside	Cardiac output exercise (twice a week)	Full-body massage (twice a month)
Calming app (2–3 times)		
10-minute afternoon nap	Stretching and mobility work (twice a week)	Acupuncture for stress (twice a month)

Phase 1: Recovery Exercise

The first step in creating a body that is resilient to stress and possesses the stamina for long-term high performance is to rebuild your aerobic system. This begins with *cardiac output exercise,* which is low-level exercise that causes the chambers of the heart to stretch, allowing more blood to be pumped with each beat, thereby providing more oxygen to meet the demands of exercise. Positive benefits from this type of training seen in our clientele include a reduction in resting heart rate and blood pressure, a reduction in fatigue buildup during high-intensity exercise, deeper sleep, enhanced resilience to stress, increased energy, increased happiness, better quality and quantity of sex, and a calmer mind.

The best time to introduce a higher volume of cardiac output exercise is during the 21-Day Reset, because this increase in movement and blood flow not only decreases stress, but also aids the lymph system in detoxification, enhancing the benefits of the Reset nutrition program. We are not using this type of training for fat loss; we are using it along with the Reset to remove all the roadblocks that are keeping long-term fat loss from happening.

RECOVERY EXERCISE GUIDELINES		
Frequency	**Duration**	**Exertion, Heart Rate (bpm)**
3–5 days per week	20–45 minutes	4/10, 120–140

SAMPLE EXERCISES FOR RECOVERY EXERCISE
Walking or jogging in nature
Walking or jogging on a treadmill
Using an elliptical machine
Doing sled pulls
Using an Airdyne bike
Swimming
Rowing

Note: You can choose one exercise for the duration or combine several for the total time. The goal is to remain at an exertion level of 4/10 or keep your heart rate in the 120–140 beats-per-minute zone for the entire time.

PERCEIVED EXERTION SCALE	
10	Maximal
9	Extremely Hard
8	Really Hard
7	Hard
6	Difficult
5	Challenging
4	Moderate
3	Easy
2	Really Easy
1	Resting

RECOVERY EXERCISE WORKOUTS		
Example 1: Using One Exercise		
Exercise	**Duration**	**Exertion, Heart Rate (bpm)**
Walking or jogging in nature	5-minute warm-up	2/10, 100–120
	30 minutes	4/10, 120–140
	5-minute cool-down	2/10, 100–120

Note: Walking or jogging in nature is my favorite choice of recovery exercise. There is something very powerful and calming about doing your recovery exercise workouts out in nature. I highly recommend you use nature to your advantage during your recovery workouts.

RECOVERY EXERCISE WORKOUTS *Example 2: Using Multiple Exercises*		
Exercise	**Duration**	**Exertion, HR (bpm)**
Elliptical (warm-up)	5 minutes	2/10, 100–120
Airdyne bike	10 minutes	4/10, 120–140
Rowing machine	10 minutes	4/10, 120–140
Sled pulls	10 minutes	4/10, 120–140
Elliptical (cool-down)	5 minutes	2/10, 100–120

If you are someone who struggles with the idea of only doing recovery exercise and not training hard for a couple of weeks, here are some guidelines for you. Remember, the people who get the best results are the ones who reduce their high-intensity exercise during the Stark Naked 21-Day Metabolic Reset.

HIGH-INTENSITY EXERCISE GUIDELINES		
Frequency	**Duration**	**Exertion, Heart Rate (bpm)**
0–2 days max	20–45 minutes	7/10 max, 130–170* max
* The HR will go up and down with effort and rest periods. The goal is to have your heart rate be in this range for the majority of the workout.		

SAMPLE EXERCISE PROGRAMS FOR HIGH-INTENSITY TRAINING
Lifting weights (avoid going to failure and no accentuated eccentric training)
Cardio intervals
Spin class
Modified strongman—sled pulls, prowler pushes, farmer walks, tire flips, etc.

Play Is the Ultimate Exercise!

When we were younger, most of us loved exercise, even if we didn't know it.

Why?

Because exercise was disguised as "play."

As children, play was our reward, not our punishment. Ask a child what his or her favorite subject in school is, and you'll likely get the reply, "Recess." My son sure loves it. Sadly, it's rare that I speak with adults who tell me their favorite part of the day is their exercise. Most loathe going to the gym, but force themselves to do it, because they think it will help them look and feel better.

As we age, we view play as childish and frown upon it. Many have forgotten how to play. That's so sad, especially when you start reading the research on the impact play can have on adults' lives. Avoid play if you want to be less effective at work, depressed, unhappy, unmotivated, lack creativity, and a poor problem solver. However, play has been shown to be one of the most powerful tools for an enhanced life. Research continually validates play as a powerful tool to boost our mood, motivation, creativity, and problem-solving skills and even help reduce our weight.

At a Driven for Life leadership retreat I attended, one of the core areas of focus was the power of play. Earlier in the day we had completed a team challenge that took my group 11 minutes. After the challenge the retreat trainers had us play a really fun game unrelated to the challenge. There was lots of laughing and activity during the game. Once the game ended, which I can proudly say my team won, we were allowed to strategize as a group about the earlier challenge with the option of redoing it. The creative juices flowing through the group were amazing. After rethinking our strategy, we were able to complete the challenge in 16 seconds. This exercise taught me that play is a powerful tool for creativity that few of us take advantage of.

We do not stop playing because we grow old;
we grow old because we stop playing.
—GEORGE BERNARD SHAW

Over the years I have found ways to get creative with exercise to keep me motivated. Since I spend most of my days in the gym, sometimes the last thing I want to do is spend even more time in the gym, away from my wife and kids, to get in a personal workout.

My solution? I play with my kids! They are little Energizer bunnies and have the stamina to play until daddy has to give up. I love this kind of time together so much that I have set up our home life around creative, fun play.

One of my favorite games is freeze tag with Nerf guns. The game works like this. We start by opening all the doors and gates around the house. We even open the windows. The goal is for me to chase the kids and their friends and try to shoot them with a Nerf dart. Talk about insane conditioning—I am dripping with sweat by the time we finish playing. The best part is hearing my kids scream with joy and laugh as I am in hot pursuit. We play for hours at a time, getting lost in the fun.

It's so rewarding for me in my relationship with my kids. It's exercise that is as far from punishment as you can get, yet it's super-beneficial for my body and my children's bodies. We also play all forms of sports together. I have even tried to mimic their acrobatics training on the grass with them. When was the last time you tried to do a cartwheel? They're so much fun, but wow, they're a lot tougher to do at forty! Yet another reason to keep trying!

Play can be tough at first, so here are some fun ideas to get you started:

Go bowling.

Throw a Frisbee at the park.

Shoot baskets.

Play on the playground at a park.

Go paintballing.

Go paddle boarding (warning: start in a bay or lake; it's tough on the open ocean).

Hike in nature.

Play tag with your kids.

Host a game night at your house. I recommend Hedbanz, as it gets really animated.

Twirl hula hoops.

Go to Chuck E. Cheese's to play games (not eat the pizza!).

Build a fort.

Have a dance party.

One of the greatest tips I received on playing with my children came from one of my clients, Dr. Daniel G. Amen, the "Brain Doctor" and *New York Times* bestselling author of *Change Your Brain, Change Your Life*. He taught me the most powerful thing I can do with my kids is to play with them every week *on their terms*. The structure is simple. I give them my undivided attention, and they take the lead. I simply become part of their game and don't dictate or correct anything. It's so much fun to be absorbed into your child's creativity and imaginary worlds. The connection you experience during these times with your kids is unbelievable. Over the years I've been everything from a pirate at sea, to a ninja in training, to a frog jumping lily pads.

I believe in the power of fun so much that I've even incorporated it into my live training seminars, where I use the game Smack Fu to engage play and wake up my audiences. Smack Fu uses a simple toy that is shaped like a dart with feathers on it. You hit it back and forth to each other, trying to keep it in the air rather than letting it hit the floor. Think volleyball without a net. It's so much fun to watch a group of serious CEOs lighten up by playing Smack Fu in the boardroom.

Creative play is a vital part of a healthy life. Stop taking life so seriously and start adding some fun back in. If you hate the gym, don't go. Replace it with play. People will notice. One of my clients, a professional NFL player I hadn't seen for a while, texted me after a training session asking what I had been doing different, because I looked younger, happier, leaner, and stronger than I had in the past two years. He said he wanted some of my "new secret sauce." I texted him back, "I stopped beating myself up in the gym and started focusing on relaxing more and engaging more in the ultimate form of exercise—*play*."

Reduce intense exercise during the Reset. You need an off-season!

10

Tap into Your Ninja Motivation and Stark Naked Mindset

L ET'S FACE IT, we all want to look better, have more energy, or spend more time with family, yet year after year we continually fail at our attempts to stick with and obtain these goals.

I get it! Change is tough. In fact, dealing with change is, I believe, one of our greatest internal struggles. A lot of you already know the changes you need to make to reach that new level of health and wellness, but you can't seem to make a dent in getting there, or you attempt it for a short time, but then fall right back into your former ways. It's true that old habits die hard.

Sadly, most people don't understand what stimulates permanent change. You might think it has to do with willpower, but science has proven willpower is like a muscle. After a while, it fatigues, leaving you vulnerable, especially later in the day. (Hint: that's why most people blow their diets in the evening. I will teach you how to use that to your advantage later in this program.)

Here's some interesting news. When it comes to change, willpower is not the solution. The answer for change lies much deeper inside you.

I have spent a lot of time studying change and have come to the realization that the most powerful creator of change is something I unknowingly used on my father when I was just three years old. My dad was a smoker. For the first few years of my young life, he fought hard to quit. He was constantly trying new strategies, but they never created lasting change. He tried everything from the patch to hypnotization, but nothing was successful in helping my father quit for good. That is, until one day I came across a pack of my dad's cigarettes and, wanting to be just like my dad, I put one in my mouth and pretended I was smoking. When my dad walked into the room and saw the cigarette hanging from my lips, his heart sank. That's all it took to keep my father from ever smoking again.

From that point on, my parents decided to focus on being healthy examples for their children. I remember sitting next to my mom's exercise mat at the community center while she did Jazzercise and being mesmerized watching my dad and his buddies lift weights at the gym. I have been hooked on exercise ever since.

When it comes to change, it's not enough to commit to making the change for yourself, because you will almost always fail. To be lasting, change must be made for those you love the most.

Just as my father witnessed me as a three-year-old with a cigarette hanging out my little mouth, you are doing things right now that those you love the most are picking up as habits. You are not talking about them, but it's sinking into their consciousness, and they are more than likely slowly developing the same unhealthy habits you're struggling with. If you currently have children, take a few minutes and observe their behavior. You might be surprised at what you see. For most of you, it will be a scary realization, but one you can start to do something about right now.

By the way, if you don't have children, you're not off the hook.

Look around at those you love the most. Do you notice any similarities in habits?

It's amazing how powerful our influence is when we do things for those we love—whether positive or negative. We will move mountains for our families, yet when it comes to doing something positive for ourselves, something as simple as eating more vegetables, that thing becomes our immovable mountain. Most of us who are caring for others tend to put those others first in our lives, leaving our own needs for last. We feel as though we just don't have the time to take care of ourselves, especially with so many demands being placed on us today.

A CEO client who has lost over 60 pounds and has totally rejuvenated his life following the Stark Naked 21-Day Metabolic Reset asked me to speak to his executive team about this concept. When I finished the talk, he came up to me with a look of absolute sadness on his face.

"My nineteen-year-old daughter is home visiting from college, and I was really bothered watching her rifle through the pantry looking for unhealthy snacks every night before she went to bed. After hearing you speak, I now realize she learned that from me! That was my comfort blanket to help me deal with stress. I can't believe I caused that," he said.

"I know how hard it is to realize this, but you should be proud that you have changed your messaging. She now sees how great you look, how much energy you have, and how happy you are. She's subconsciously watching the new you. It's critical to just keep walking your path. It will rub off on her! I promise," I assured him.

My client was amazed how his habits had influenced hers, because they had never spoken about it. She just seemed to pick them up. Unfortunately that's how it works; our actions speak so much louder than our words.

Don't think you can live one way, but tell your loved ones to live another. You must live your example!

Ninja Motivation

Every year I sit down with each of my kids to help them set individual goals and dreams to pursue. I started them with this type of goal setting at the youngest possible age as a way of helping them set up their year with something to strive for. You can never be too young for that. Two years ago, my daughter, Isabel, who was just five at the time, hit me with a left hook on the chin with her reality.

The night before we did her goals, I took her with me to sit in on a talk I was doing with a basketball team about health and performance. I downloaded a new game on my iPad to keep her occupied while I spoke. During my talk she sat in the corner, appearing to be fully engaged in the new game, so I figured, like most kids, she probably heard nothing that came out of her father's mouth.

The next morning Isabel and I sat down to work on her goals. We write them out together, but I always make it a point to let my children choose their own goals, as I want them to pursue what they want, not what I want for them. Her first two goals were great:

Goal 1: I can read a book.

Goal 2: I can do a handstand.

I loved how she innately wrote them in a form that seemed to say she had already accomplished them. Goal 3, however, threw me for a bit of a loop.

Goal 3: I drink more water.

Huh? Where did that come from? When I saw that on her list, my initial response as a sometimes oblivious father was to think she was being a little lazy and not really putting a great deal of thought into her third goal.

"Honey, your goals are great. I really like goals 1 and 2. We can really track your progress and work toward reaching them, but I am a little confused by goal number 3. Why did you decide that drinking more water should be your third major goal this year?"

"Daddy, I heard you talk to that basketball team last night, and you told them if they wanted to be better athletes and healthier, they needed to drink more water. Well, I want to be a ninja when I grow up. That means I need to be a better athlete and healthier, so I need to drink more water like those basketball players. I also see you and Mommy drinking water all the time, so it must be really important."

Her response was beautiful. Admittedly, I was floored at first, because I couldn't believe she heard me speaking to the basketball team. I also couldn't believe she was taking her father's advice. Isabel proceeded to quote all of my major talking points from the night before. I had almost missed an amazing opportunity to realize that I am a living example for my daughter—in a positive way. Not only had she heard my advice; she was paying close attention to and watching the actions of her mother and me. I have saved that year's list of goals as a constant reminder of what I now call *ninja motivation*.

Ninjas are lethal, yet you never see them coming. They're similar to our lifestyle habits, because they can silently enhance or destroy the lives of those we love the most. How is your ninja motivation affecting those around you whom you love the most?

If, like my father, you're not happy with how you are silently affecting the lives of your loved ones, now is the perfect time to change. It was my dad's ninja motivation that led me to write this book. Without it, I wouldn't have had the exposure to health and fitness or the desire to dedicate my life to helping others find their inner ninja!

The greatest gift you can give those around you is to live the change you want to see in them. Live the lifestyle habits you want them to pick up and enjoy in their lives. I can't imagine anyone who would want their loved ones to require a constant intake of caffeine to have enough energy to survive their days or push their children into a pattern of not sleeping enough by constantly telling them sleep is for the weak.

The majority of our referrals at Stark don't come from people who

Ninja Motivation Exercise for Success

To truly be successful and create lasting change, you must take a good look at how your ninja motivation is affecting those you love the most. Get a pen and piece of paper and take some time to answer these few questions. Do not think you are doing this for yourself and no one else. That may be enough to get you started, but it won't keep you in the change game long-term.

1. Whom do I love the most in this world? List three to five people for whom you want to be a powerful positive ninja motivator.
2. How is my lifestyle currently affecting these people? List five things you are doing that make you a positive ninja motivator. List five things you are doing that make you a negative ninja motivator.
3. What does my new lifestyle look like? List three lifestyle goals associated with your new ninja motivation that will enhance the lives of those you love the most. (Example: Sleeping 7 hours a night for great natural energy, leading to a more youthful and energetic me all day long.)

have been told by our happy and satisfied clients how great we are, but rather from people who have witnessed the positive changes in those people and asked about how those changes came about. They then come to us to get those results for themselves.

Our clients are using their ninja motivation to improve the lives of their family and friends. Trust me—they are watching!

Change Is Hard!

In 2013 I had the incredible opportunity to work with my first SWAT team, providing nutrition and supplementation strategies to help optimize their energy, sleep, and performance. It was such an honor and a challenge, because these are some tough-minded individuals who are resistant to things they don't know or aren't familiar with. I met with them at their regular training grounds. In between testing and working with them, I sometimes got to watch them do their SWAT training exercises, clearing mock houses, practicing target shooting, and so on. Sometimes I got to play the bad guy they were hunting down!

One situation took place in a huge studio with different movie sets. I was the bad guy hiding in an office setting, while the SWAT team came to find me. I was hiding behind a door and remember looking through the crack, right into the eyes of an ex-Navy SEAL as he had me locked in his rifles sites. The intense, focused look in his eyes genuinely scared me.

After several months of training together, they decided that if I wanted to stick around, it was time for me to experience one of their physical workouts with them. I needed to keep their respect, so naturally I accepted their invitation, knowing I was in for an ass kicking. The 1½-hour drive to the workout site was gut-wrenching. I had no idea what to expect, but there was one certainty: it was going to be hell. I went into the physical challenge with two major goals. First, no matter what challenges I faced, I was going to finish. Second, I was not going to come in last place.

Eleven reps into the workout I knew I was in serious trouble. The workout started with 25 pull-ups. The first 10 had to be strict, but after that you could move into CrossFit-style kipping pull-ups that generated a lot of momentum in the movement, making them a lot easier. The only problem was that I had never done a kipping pull-up.

I was able to keep up for the first 10 reps, but then the team took off flying through kipping reps while I struggled to finish. Right out of the gate I fell into last place.

We moved on to what felt like endless repetitions of full-body exercises using heavy sandbags as weights combined with long runs carrying the sandbags on our shoulders. Halfway through these combos, my world started closing in on me. My whole body and mind screamed, *"Stop!"*

My legs were becoming numb. With every step I took, I felt as though I was one step shy of crumbling to the ground. My lungs were burning, and nausea had set in and taken over my body. I had never experienced anything like this.

I had so much respect for these guys coming into this. I didn't want to fail them; if I quit, they would never look at me the same again. I dug deep and repeated my personal motto, "Just keep going. It will eventually end. All pain ends sooner or later."

At the 14th minute of the nonstop high-intensity exercise, I faced two options: to finish or pass out. Those were the only two options I would consider to make the pain stop.

I wanted to maintain my honor with these men I looked up to so much. I pushed myself and completed the sandbag exercise, remaining runs, and 25 more agonizing pull-ups before I finally crossed the finish line. It took every last ounce of my energy to complete that 25th pull-up, but I found a way to finish.

Okay, I'll admit that I finished 10 minutes behind the top guy, but hey, I still finished! And as promised, I didn't finish last.

This 24 minutes of straight high-intensity exercise almost ended my life, but once the pain was over, I was so proud of myself for digging deep and pushing myself beyond what I believed I was ever capable of.

One thing I have learned over the years is that we are capable of far more than we believe. Too many of us set up mental boundaries and give up early on things without ever really trying. We give up before we even attempt them, because we convince ourselves we don't have what it takes.

One common area I see people hold themselves back in is their health and fitness. I hear the craziest excuses about why people won't try to eat healthier or exercise. Most of them are basically bullsh-t. You can do whatever you set your mind to.

Here are some strategies like those I used during my workout with the SWAT team to help you *thrive* when you have to push through tough times.

Thrive Strategy 1: Focus on small things.

At times, focusing on the big picture can be daunting and over-whelming. How do you overcome this kind of challenge? Merely break it down and focus on one small step at a time. During the workout with the SWAT team, I focused on simply taking each next step. Life is all about one baby step at a time, and that strategy got me to the finish line.

When it comes to the Stark Naked 21-Day Metabolic Reset, you might find yourself dealing with hunger the first 3 to 5 days on the plan. Instead of thinking about how many days you have left on the plan or on the foods you can't eat, focus on reaching your next meal without cheating! Set a goal that you will not contemplate giving up until after you have eaten your next meal. It's that simple. Surviving and thriving come from taking small continuous steps, not one huge leap.

Thrive Strategy 2: Never forget your ninja motivation.

Who are you doing this for? When times get tough, picture those people in your mind. They will give you the deep motivation to take another step forward. There have been many times in my life that I have had to close my eyes and picture my wife and children to help motivate me.

Recently, I have been given the opportunity to create a full-immersion destination retreat focused on the Stark Naked 21-Day Metabolic Reset in Belize. During the 5-to-7-day getaway, people will be disconnected from the world, so they can focus on dramatically enhancing their health. They say this location is the closest thing to the Garden of Eden on earth. It's such an amazing opportunity for me, my business, the people whose lives I want to enhance, and my family. The drawback is that my investors want the plan formulated and launched ASAP!

This is a huge opportunity and dream come true, but it's creating enormous stress in my life, because it means I have to take time away from the things I love and need the most for balance and well-being. To help keep me centered and focused, I keep pictures of my wife and kids all over, on my desk, the wallpaper on my phone, iPad, laptop, and so on. Seeing their smiling faces helps to keep me going when I am tired and frustrated, as I know this retreat will bring life-changing experiences for all of us.

I am the kind of guy who needs and enjoys constant reminders of those I love, especially when the pressure builds up. Sometimes, I will admit, I'm tempted to throw in the towel and give up. But when I see my family, even if it's just in my mind, it helps me look past the current obstacles and push forward.

Thrive Strategy 3: The pain will eventually come to an end.

In the movie *Unbroken,* the main character, Louie, suffers being lost at sea and the horrors of prisoner-of-war camps, but has a resiliency that is incredibly inspirational. He represents the epitome of what we as humans are capable of enduring. His brother gave him the best advice for survival, "If you can take it, you can make it."

That is exactly how I have chosen to live my life too. Although I haven't endured the kind of hardship he did as a prisoner of war, I understand that as long as I don't give up, the pain eventually ends—and it always does.

This way of thinking helped me survive my freshman year of college. I grew up loving sports. I especially excelled at baseball, eventually earning a spot on a college baseball team. My freshman year, the coach at the four-year college I was attending decided it would be a better idea if I played at a junior college for the year and then come back, instead of sitting on the bench for the year as a red-shirt freshman.

I agreed. I would much rather have played than sat.

That decision was one of the worst choices I ever made. However, it was also one of the best character-building experiences I have endured. The coach of the junior college I attended was young and, for reasons I will never understand, had it in for me. It was his mission to break me. I played baseball because I loved the game; he viewed baseball as a way to prove you're a man. Every day I had to deal with his negativity. One day he actually challenged me to a fight after I questioned him about what it was going to take for me to get more playing time.

We all experience people like this in life at one time or another—a horrible boss, a negative friend, the wrong girlfriend or boyfriend. Many of you have even known a coach like this as well.

People like this eventually fizzle out. One day, you will no longer have to deal with them, and the pain goes away. No matter what, you have to keep getting out of bed every morning, and you can't let them beat you. Knowing the pain would eventually end helped push me forward, forcing me to keep going.

When I opened my first gym in 2004, I was so financially strapped I had to sleep on a buddy's couch and shower at the gym, because I couldn't afford to pay the bills for the gym *and* rent my own living space. I believed in my training philosophies and wanted to share them with the world my way, but, man, it was a struggle to establish myself in Southern California, where there are gyms on every street corner. So early on, there were many days when I had no idea how I was going to find the money to pay the rent on the gym and keep the lights on. But as long as I didn't give up, I knew that pain would eventually go away—and eventually it did.

Those early struggles have given me the resiliency and character to fight through tough times whenever they arise. And believe me, they do. Tough times are a part of everyone's life. Understanding that the pain will eventually end is where we should focus, not on how bad it hurts. This belief system still gets me out of bed even today when

I am mentally and physically fatigued and I am second-guessing myself and my ability to be an agent of change.

Here's the bottom line: *the start of the Reset is tough*. There is no doubt about it. But you have survived much worse things than this in your life. For the next 21 days I want you to step up for yourself and everyone you love and simply be *all in* all the time!

When I was a kid, my father used to tell me every morning, "Every day you are either getting better or getting worse, but you are never staying the same, so do something today that makes you better." I pass that same advice on to you, but I want to add one more thing: "Change your life and you literally change the world." You will never understand the true power of your ninja motivation, but your simple change will have a ripple effect for generations to come.

> For the next 21 days, I want you to step up for yourself and everyone you love and simply be *all in* all the time!

▶ PART FOUR

THE STARK NAKED 21-DAY METABOLIC RESET

11

Phase 1

The Stark Naked 21-Day Metabolic Reset

TIME TO RESET AND REBOOT!

By now I hope you understand that it's not been your lack of effort or something you've been consciously doing wrong that got you where you are today.

You've put in the right amount of effort. You've had enough will-power! You've exercised—likely more than you needed to. You've probably deprived yourself of the foods you needed. You've certainly done all of the right things, hoping to look, feel, and perform better—and despite everything, you don't!

Honestly, it's not your fault!

Your metabolism is simply b-r-o-k-e-n! You need to bring it back online—hit the reset button. Shut down the system and reboot, so you can feel great, look amazing, and finally perform with the boundless energy you've been looking for.

As you have finally discovered, it has likely been your overzealous quest for health, your ignorance about your liver, and eating the wrong foods for you, even *healthy* foods, that have left you looking and feeling the way you do.

As of today, there will be no more trying to force change. There will only be your acceptance that your body needs a break and your willingness to give it one.

Oh, hey. Check your cell phone.

What?

It's frozen?

You can't check your messages?

Get your e-mails?

Texts?

Sh-t!

What would you do if that really happened?

C'mon, be honest.

If you're like most people, you'd likely turn the thing off and reboot it.

It's called a *reset*.

Get it?

Why would you panic over your phone and not do the same over your health?

Imagine it this way. You and I are racing cars against each other in a 500-mile race. You can choose whatever car you want for our race. My favorite car is the 1967 Ford Mustang Shelby GT500 Fastback, the same car that is Nicholas Cage's nemesis in the movie *Gone in 60 Seconds*. The race we are in is all about performance, so make sure you choose a seriously high-performing car.

Got it?

Okay.

Here we go!

We are off!

Everything is going smoothly! We're neck in neck in the early stages. We spend the first few hundred miles fairly even, until suddenly a light starts flashing on my dashboard.

Uh-oh. It's the gas light warning me that I am running out of fuel. I am forced to make a pit stop to refuel my car.

My momentary lapse gives you a chance to pull ahead, until you notice your fuel light blinking. That little voice in your head begins telling you that you can't stop now. If you pull off, I will catch up to you. You convince yourself to push through and just ignore the warning sign. Despite the obvious flashing light, you push the pedal to the metal and go flying right past the pit row. You are brimming with excitement because your lead has grown so much. You believe there is no way I will ever catch up until . . . *clunk!* Your car jerks hard a few times, and then your engine dies. You're out of gas!

The smart solution would be to refuel, but you pride yourself on working harder than everyone else, and that little voice in your head continues to tell you that you cannot afford to circle back, so you jump out and start pushing your car as hard as you can toward the finish line, believing your hard work and perseverance will overcome the lack of gas in your tank and, somehow, you will still win this race. Obviously you have no chance. The reality is you will never even finish the race.

It's a silly story, but that's exactly what we are doing with our bodies when we ignore the warning signs that something is broken and needs to be fixed. We think we are invincible or can sacrifice in ways others can't, because we are high achievers. But we can't. No one can. Eventually, that tank runs out of gas. And no matter how hard you push the car, it will never cross the finish line.

Professional athletes are experts at this, because the majority of them take downtime during the off-season to recover from all the hard work and stress they put their body through during the regular season. The professional athletes we work with at Stark aren't allowed to intensely train in the gym when they are on mandatory rest. They are only allowed to do recovery exercises (as discussed earlier, in Chapter 9). They can get massages, spend quality time with their families, get physical therapy for the beat-up areas of their bodies, and give themselves a much-needed break. When they do this, they come back with renewed energy and find themselves ready to train harder and with the chance of less injury. As a result, their progress preparing for the new season is always amazing.

As busy high achievers, most of us never take a break—from anything! Maybe, just maybe, you'll take a vacation, but a recent poll showed that Americans take the least amount of vacation time compared to people in all the other countries in the world.

Everyone needs a break from time to time. If you want the stamina to finish life strong, you will treat this advice as if your life depends on it—because it does.

I recently started working with a client who is a senior PR executive for a major corporation. In some instances, being a public-relations executive can be as stressful as being an emergency-room doctor! To reach the position of senior executive in a large organization, you must be a serious high achiever.

When I first met my client, it was obvious her body had fought the good fight until age forty. But all of a sudden her body started giving out on her. Over the course of the next five years, during which she lived her life exactly the same way she always had, stress began to win the battle. Her body weight began to increase as her energy tanked and lethargy kicked in. She just couldn't keep up the same pace, even though she was doing all of the same things she had done throughout the years to stay in shape and look great. Intuitively she quickly realized something wasn't right. She understood if she didn't make some changes, not only would she not have the stamina to finish out her career; she could get very sick.

This client was very open and honest about her health and future. She had heard a talk I gave to a group of overachieving executives on how fitness masks health. Like most of my clients, she was someone who believed if 30 minutes of exercise was good for her, 90 minutes was better.

Sound like anyone you know? She was the driver unwilling to pull off the track for gas.

This woman pulled into the Brad Davidson repair shop out of gas, with two flat tires, the emergency brake stuck on, and a dragging muffler. She had been pushing her car around for years, believing she was performing at her highest level. After years of taking, the time had come to give back to her body. Leadership consultant Robin Sharma said it best: "Peak performance without strategic refueling leads to enduring depletion."

The Stark Naked 21-Day Metabolic Reset is my gift to you and your metabolism. It's the strategic refueling your metabolism and body are in dire need of.

I want to help you have this breakthrough, but it's time for a new strategy. It's *recovery*—not a willingness to work harder than the next person—that enables the highest performers long-term. Recovery is the true art that enhances performance at the highest level. I know this is hard to believe, and that is why I am challenging you to take only 21 of your (on average) 27,375 days here on earth to test this theory.

So instead of hitting the gym every day, you're going to do things to relax along with following the program, and for some of you that will be harder than giving up some of your favorite foods for three weeks. You're going to cut back on your exercise. You are only allowed two 45-minute high-intensity exercise sessions a week max during the first 21 days. You can do recovery exercise like leisurely walking every day, but you will need to dramatically reduce your high-intensity exercise, and that's going to feel strange at first. If you are really tired, I would highly recommend doing only the recovery exercise discussed in Chapter 9.

Believe it or not, cutting out the self-imposed demand to do and be busy all the time will have a profound impact on your body and well-being. I'm giving you the green light to sit on the couch and relax. Your metabolism, appearance, sex drive, performance level, and general well-being all need this. In fact, they're crying out for it. This is your free pass, so take it.

Why the Stark Naked 21-Day Metabolic Reset Works

Having worked with thousands of clients on this very program, I have witnessed firsthand the challenges they faced on a daily basis to make it through, both mentally and physically. Although the eating portion of the plan isn't necessarily "hard," the general mindset of most people going into it is that it's going to be. To overcome that immediate perception, the program is designed to help improve your likelihood of success. Willpower is like a muscle: *the more it's used, the more it fatigues.* It has been scientifically proven that a person loses willpower and becomes more likely to make poor decisions as the day goes on. I've watched this happen with my clients at Stark. Who hasn't grabbed a midnight snack or something at the airport late in the day that they later regretted?

To combat declining willpower, the Stark Naked 21-Day Metabolic Reset places the toughest choices, like avoiding carbs, early in the day, when your willpower is strongest, and the easier choices later in the day, when your willpower is weakening, dramatically increasing the likelihood of success. By loosening the noose at night and allowing you the freedom of carbohydrates at dinner and a bedtime snack, this plan virtually ensures success. You won't fall prey to weak willpower.

The Eleven Lifestyle Modifications for the Stark Naked 21-Day Metabolic Reset

Now that you know why you're here, it's time to understand the outline of the game for the next 21 days. The following are the eleven core lifestyle strategies of the Reset. Follow these strategies and stick with the plan, and I promise you will see remarkable results. You can't cheat on *any* of these, or it will impact your results. Any deviation will mean the difference between success or failure. Hey, I'm just the messenger. If you don't like what you see in the mirror, don't break the mirror. Change the reflection!

The first four modifications include strategies to reduce your stress load and get better control of your cortisol, the next three include removing all of the unneeded sources of stress on your liver, and the final four are to help you get the most from your diet.

1. Hydrate. For the next 21 days, water is going to be your new BFF. You will need to drink one-half of your body weight in ounces of water a day. For example, if you weigh 150 pounds, you will need to drink 75 ounces of water every day. It won't be easy, but it will be worth it. Water, vitally important to the human body, helps reduce cortisol and really aids in the detoxification process. Yes, you will be going to the bathroom more than usual in the beginning, but the frequency ought to slow down after the first few days.

If it doesn't you, can try adding minerals to your water to help improve your body's ability to absorb the water into your cells. A high-stress lifestyle can severely deplete these minerals, preventing your body from absorbing the water, which creates a flushing effect. What this means is that you drink water and it essentially flushes right out in your urine without doing its job, leaving you dehydrated. It's a very common reason so many people complain of constantly having to go to the bathroom after drinking more water. I personally like adding ConcenTrace minerals to my water. You can find those at most health-food and supplement stores or online.

2. Sleep 7 to 9 hours a night every night. Remember, almost all animals on earth need sleep. The only exceptions are those lacking complex mental functions like jellyfish and flatworms. The more complicated the brain, the more sleep a creature needs. That is why you are going to aim for 7 to 9 hours of sleep every night. I want you in bed by no later than 11:00 P.M. Sleep recharges your battery, and it's when your body goes into healing mode! If you have trouble sleeping, try some of the sleep suggestions in Chapter 8.

3. Drastically reduce your intense exercise. You can train hard for a maximum of 45 minutes 2 days per week, but it is not mandatory. Remember, less is more during your reset. You can do other forms of training, such as the recovery exercise we talked about, but it is critical that your perceived exertion during these workouts stays at 4/10. That is the level that allows you to carry on a full conversation during the workout without feeling winded or breathless. Those of you who don't adhere to this advice, who think you will outsmart me, or who *need* to hit it hard are in for a real awakening. You will *not* get the full benefit of this program. Intense exercise elevates cortisol and bogs the liver down. It will have an impact *opposite* to the one you're seeking.

4. Commit to daily acts of relaxation. Research shows that as little as 10 minutes of relaxation a day has major benefits for your body. All I am asking for is at least 10 minutes of focused relaxation each day. Anything that you find relaxing works. Some examples are meditation, focused deep breathing, reading a book, or simply taking a 10-minute catnap in the afternoon. Trust me, on days 2 and 3 it won't take much persuasion to get you to take a nap. If you have trouble meditating, try one of the apps I mentioned in Chapter 6 (also see the Resource Guide for these).

5. No coffee. Ugh! I know I am ruthless! I am a giver though, because you can have green tea for a little caffeine if you need it. Green tea is loaded with great metabolism and liver support. If you do cut out coffee and caffeine altogether, the headache and energy crash you may feel will only last for the first 3 to 5 days, after which your natural energy will emerge and every day you will feel better and better. *Push through!* It is worth it to feel that natural energy and clarity come back. It's been years since you've had it, and you might just like it.

6. No alcohol. Before your throw this book at someone or across the room, remember, it's only 21 days! Rehab is 28! If you seriously can't give up booze for 21 days, maybe you ought to be looking at

Betty Ford instead of Brad Davidson. Okay, just kidding. Here's some good news! After 21 days, I'll let you put alcohol back in your routine—if you still want it.

Truthfully, so many of my clients tell me once that they get past the first 5 days, they are amazed at how great they feel. Their energy and clarity, especially in the morning, are fantastic. People who drink alcohol, even one to three drinks a night, are impacting their sleep, sometimes wake with a slight hangover, and can be foggy the next day—often without realizing it. Habits are formed. You learn to live as if this is feeling "normal," when in fact you are impaired. Twenty-one days will shed some light on this for you as well as help you shed some pounds. I can't think of a better reason to give it up or give it a try. Stop hyperventilating! You'll be okay going 21 days without alcohol.

7. Remove refined sugar from your diet—all sources of refined sugar. If you have a sweet tooth, this may be the hardest part of the plan for you, especially for the first few days. Believe it or not, on average, most Americans consume 136 pounds of sugar a year, and about 20 percent of their calories come from sugar. That's 25 teaspoons a day! Kids are eating even more than that! Yikes!

Sugar is nothing but empty calories that are adding pounds and causing more harm than good. Worse, for some, it's as addictive as any illicit drug. The brain depends on blood glucose for its energy. Eating anything with sucrose in it can cause a variation in blood-glucose levels. If you want to stabilize those levels, eliminate, or at the very least cut way down on, your total sugar intake. For this program, eliminate all added sugars and foods that are high in refined sugar. Getting off the sugar treadmill isn't easy, but it's totally worth it.

I had a client text me 10 days into his metabolic reset that he felt as if he was getting out of an abusive relationship, because he had no idea how bad his addiction to sugar had become until he was away from it. Halfway through his reset, he suddenly realized how damaging his nutrition and stressful lifestyle were. It was crushing him.

When he finished, he said he'd never recommit to that bad relationship with his food or way of life ever again.

I want you to have the same kind of breakthrough, whether it's with sugar or the things mentioned in any of the other ten lifestyle modifications. One amazing side effect of giving up sugar is you'll begin to notice how good and flavorful other foods taste. It's not that the food tastes better; it's your taste buds coming alive! Cool, huh?

One other important note about sugar is that other sugars and sugar substitutes, such as brown sugar, saccharin, aspartame, cane juice, lactose, fruit juice sweeteners, and fructose, are not great alternatives when eliminating sugar, because they are all chemically processed sweeteners. If you must use a sweetener during the first 21 days, stevia is the only approved option.

8. Follow the list of approved foods. There are no exceptions! For the next 21 days you are going to experience my exclusive elimination-based diet that removes the most common foods people are sensitive to from your diet, based on information gathered from thousands of clients I've worked with over the years. The list of approved foods was created by finding food-induced inflammation commonalities in over 350 food-sensitivity tests (MRTs) done on high performers I personally train or trained.

If you stick with this list, your gut and allergies will thank me, and ultimately you will too. The only time I let people deviate from this is if they have an actual sensitivity lab test done—so if you know something on or off this list is specific to you, adjust accordingly. Otherwise, no cheating! Remember what you're momma always said, "Cheaters never prosper!"

9. Maximize protein and vegetable intake. This is not a deprivation diet, so don't starve yourself. The protein and vegetable serving sizes are the minimums you are allowed to eat. *You can eat as much protein and as many vegetables as you want at lunch and dinner.* (But, remember, everything has its limits, so don't go eating a 40-ounce cowboy steak thinking you aren't going to pay the price.) These foods possess the ultimate rebuilding blocks for your metabolism, so don't be shy.

10. Follow carbohydrate and fat servings exactly. This modification will mean one of two things for you: it will be either a drastic reduction or a major increase in carbohydrates for you. If it's a drastic reduction, your fatigue may last a while longer, as your body will need more time to figure out how to rely on fats rather than glucose for energy. On the other hand, if this is a drastic increase in carbs for you and you're a person who exercises all the time, then you will notice your energy will become elevated rather quickly. You will also see a nice boost in your sex drive sooner too. Lucky you!

I created this plan based on nutrient-timing philosophies, in which carbohydrates and fats really help with energy and focus during the day and then aid in improving sleep at night. Remember, recent research shows that those who eat 80 percent or more of their carbs at dinner or later actually lose more weight, specifically more fat. Although it took a lot of convincing to get my clients to eat carbs at night, those who have gone on the Stark Naked 21-Day Metabolic Reset have validated that as solid fact too.

11. Stick to three meals a day. I know this modification is still a shocker after so many years of hearing that five to six small meals a day is ideal, but I hope after reading Chapter 7, on nutritional confusion, we've built some trust and you'll be on board with me. Eating more small meals a day is actually not any better for your metabolism than eating fewer meals. There have been multiple studies substantiating it has worse results than fewer feedings each day. Try it. You might like it!

But wait . . . there's one more!

Optional Bonus Modification: Clean the toxic solvents out of your house. If you're really feeling ready to hop on the Reset train, I highly recommend taking a look at the products you are using around your house and for your personal hygiene. This is an expensive proposition, one you don't have to take on all at one time, but become aware of what you're using, breathing in, lathering up with, and slathering on and decide what you can and cannot live with. Use the SkinDeep app or www.ewg.org website to help you clean your house of toxic solvents like hygiene products, beauty products, and cleaners. Restock with safe, friendly products. Once you get the toxins out of your life, you will never want to go back to living with them again.

We Took Out the Guesswork for You

For the initial 21 days, make the commitment to stick to the following list of foods at all costs. I know it looks limited, but this elimination-style nutrition plan is one of the most powerful diet protocols I have ever seen. That's why it's at the core of this program. By removing the most common foods found to cause intolerance, the Stark Naked 21-Day Metabolic Reset helps you avoid adverse reactions to the wrong foods and is the best way to break the cycle of food addiction that is causing unnecessary stress on your body.

This plan allows you to completely remove the trigger foods, so that your body has no reason to form antibodies or develop inflammation. I know you may think you don't have issues with any foods, but trust me, you have just gotten use to the symptoms. You have become numbed to your body's response to your trigger foods. If you remove any one of these trigger foods for a while and then reintroduce that food, guess what? It will rock you!

After you have completed the initial Reset, I will teach you how to reintroduce foods back into your diet to make sure they are safe in Phase 2.

Warning! Once you've successfully completed the Reset, your energy will skyrocket and you will want to take on the world.

Understand one thing. All high achievers have a tendency to overdo things. It is a constant and sometimes vicious cycle we can fall into.

Once you start to feel better—and I promise that if you follow this plan, you are going to feel *amazing*—you will inevitably start overdoing and overachieving again. Before you know it, if you aren't careful, you will feel miserable again.

Once you fix what's broken, meaning you've successfully reset your metabolism, you must commit to taking care of yourself like the high achiever you genuinely are, so you can stay in peak condition for the rest of your life.

Are you ready to rock?

Prepare for Success

By failing to prepare, you are preparing to fail.

—BENJAMIN FRANKLIN

I am the kind of guy who needs to force myself to focus to be truly prepared. Lack of preparation is the death of success in anything. I have done the 21-Day Reset many times and have discovered some simple preparation strategies to ensure success. Above all, prep meals as much as you can ahead of time to avoid any bumps in the road and keep stress to a minimum. Breakfast and lunch are my most challenging meals, so I always make sure to prep those over the weekend and have them ready to go for the week. I'm able to prepare a Reset-friendly dinner at mealtime, but if your evenings are harried and the time when you're most likely to slip, go ahead and prep those too. Here are my favorite strategies.

Weekly Prep Strategies

Shopping and prep day: Choose one day each week to go grocery shopping and prep meals. My wife and I chose Sundays, since neither of us works on that day. It's not only quality time together; it helps set up our week for Reset success. Prep time: 1 hour to shop and 75 minutes to prep.

Breakfast prep, Stark Naked detox smoothies: Cut and divide all of the fruits and vegetables for your daily morning smoothies. Store them in small zip-top bags in your refrigerator. Each morning, all you'll need to add to your blender are the contents of a zip-top bag, your fats, and a small amount of water. It's that simple. Quick and easy, and no excuses! Prep time: 15 minutes.

Lunch prep: After preparing your detox smoothie bags, cook up a selection of meat for lunchtime. My wife and I usually cook chicken breasts, turkey patties, bison steaks, and ground wild meats. We store them in lidded glass containers in the refrigerator. We also cut up vegetables to use on salads. Prep time: 60 minutes.

Dinner prep: If you feel you need to prep dinners as well, plan on adding another 30 minutes to your total prep time.

Daily Prep Strategies

Do these at night before going to bed, so you're ready for the next day.

Warm lemon water prep: You'll begin each morning with warm lemon water. I fill the tea kettle and put in on the stove (I do it the old-fashioned way!), set out my mug, and make sure I have half of a lemon in the fridge. All I have to do when I walk out to the kitchen in the morning is turn on the stove, warm up the water, pour it into the mug, and squeeze the lemon in. Prep time: 2 minutes.

Cranberry juice cocktail prep: In a 32-ounce water bottle, combine 4 ounces of unsweetened cranberry juice (not from concentrate) and 28 ounces of water. Store in the fridge until your midmorning cocktail. Prep time: 3 minutes.

Lunch prep: To a lidded glass container, add a large bed of salad greens and any precut vegetables from your weekly prep day. Place your choice of meat from your weekly prep day on top of the salad. For the required serving of fat, dress the salad with olive oil or add avocado. Season to taste. Store in the refrigerator overnight. Prep time: 5 minutes.

A Typical Morning

Okay! It's as simple as that!

By preparing for a little over an hour each week and 10 minutes before bed each night, you can be completely ready for the week and start each day stress free. You can get out the door each morning in just five easy steps:

Step 1: Wake up.

Step 2: Heat water for your lemon water and drink.

Step 3: Get ready for work or the rest of your day.

Step 4: Throw your zip-top smoothie produce, water, and approved fats into the blender, blend, and drink.

Step 5: Grab your lunch and cranberry juice cocktail from the fridge on the way out the door.

Approved Foods

Okay, enough with the success strategies! Let's get to what you've been waiting for. Without further ado—drumroll, please—here are your approved foods for the next 21 days.

PHASE 1 APPROVED FOODS
Proteins
Eggs
Poultry (chicken, turkey, duck, ostrich, Cornish game hen)
Pork
All fish except salmon and shellfish

Wild game meats (buffalo, bison, boar, venison, antelope, duck)
Full-fat cottage cheese (only allowed as the before-bed snack)
Fats
Coconut oil
Olive oil
Macadamia nut oil
Walnut oil
Avocado oil
Seeds (sesame, flax, chia, hemp, pumpkin, and sunflower seeds)
Heavy whipping cream
Organic butter and ghee
Avocado
Unsweetened canned coconut milk
Unsweetened almond milk (only allowed in the morning smoothie)
Cashews and pecans (only allowed as the before-bed snack)
Carbohydrates
Rice (all types)
All potatoes except white potatoes (sweet potatoes, yams, red potatoes, purple potatoes)
Quinoa
Gluten-free pasta (no cornstarch)
Gluten-free oats
Vegetables
All vegetables except carrots, beets, peas, corn, and broccoli
Fruits
All fruits except bananas, grapes, blueberries, and grapefruit
Herbs and Spices
All herbs and spices
Beverages
Water
Green tea
Herbal teas
Unsweetened cranberry juice (not from concentrate)

Meals and Serving Sizes

Now let's take a look at what each day will look like for the next 21 days.

PHASE 1 DAILY OUTLINE	
Hydration	
Number of ounces of water that equals half your body weight throughout the day (includes cranberry juice cocktails)	
Upon Waking	
6 ounces warm water with juice from ½ lemon	
Breakfast (within 1 hour of waking)	
Stark Naked detox smoothie (see recipes, pp. 222–29)	
Green tea (in addition to the smoothie)	
Mid-Morning Snack	
As much of the cranberry juice cocktail (4 ounces unsweetened cranberry juice, not from concentrate, mixed with 28 ounces water) as you'd like now; finish the rest between meals throughout the day	
Lunch	
Men	2 servings protein, 2 servings vegetables, 2 servings fat*
Women	1 serving protein, 2 servings vegetables, 1 serving fat*
Mid-Afternoon Snack	
Green tea	
Dinner	
Men	2 servings protein, 2 servings vegetables, 2 servings fat, 2 servings carbs*
Women	1 serving protein, 2 servings vegetables, 1 serving fat, 1 serving carbs*
Before-Bed Snack	
1 serving fruit and ½ cup full-fat cottage cheese, or a handful of cashews or pecans	
Note: Portions of protein and vegetables are the minimum requirements for each meal. You can consume as much protein and vegetables as needed at each meal to keep you satiated. Portions of fats, carbohydrates, and fruits cannot be changed.	

PHASE 1 SERVING SIZES	
Protein	1 serving = 3 ounces uncooked meat (about the size of a deck of cards), 2 whole eggs
Vegetables	1 serving = 1 cup raw
Fat	1 serving = 1 tablespoon oil, butter, or heavy whipping cream, ½ avocado, ¼ cup seeds
Carbohydrates	1 serving = 1 cup *cooked*
Fruit	1 serving = ½ cup

Daily Steps for Success

Here are the six daily steps in the program that help ensure your success and create long-term change.

Step 1: Warm Lemon Water

You will start your day by drinking warm lemon water to enhance liver detoxification and improve digestion. Warm lemon water also helps increase energy, strengthen the immune system, and improve the quality of the skin.

Step 2: Stark Naked Detox Smoothie

Our exclusive detox green smoothies are a favorite among our clients for breakfast. They are a great way to get a lot of nutrients into the body fast. Plus, they are superfilling and taste great.

We all know the importance of fruits and vegetables, but very few of us consume anywhere near the recommended 9 servings a day. Blending the fruits and vegetables into a smoothie makes them easier to digest, preventing the bloating and intestinal irritation that usually accompanies increased fruit and vegetable intake. I prefer blending to juicing, because the fiber is not removed from the fruits and vegetables when you blend. Fiber improves the quality and regularity of bowel movements, removes toxins from the body, stabilizes blood sugar, and lowers cholesterol.

Green vegetable-based smoothies also have an alkalizing effect on the body, neutralizing and eliminating excess acid that can cause indigestion and other digestive issues. The most rewarding benefit of these green smoothies is improved blood flow. Better blood circulation leads to more action in the bedroom. As Dr. Daniel Amen says, "What's good for the heart, is good for the brain, is good for the genitals."

Step 3: Unsweetened Cranberry Juice

I will confess that developing a taste for unsweetened cranberry juice may not be pleasant at first, but you do get used to it. It is very important to stay away from cranberry juice from concentrate, as it is loaded with high-fructose corn syrup. This type of sugar places a heavy burden on the liver, and we are trying to reduce the stress on the liver, not add to it. I learned about the power of cranberry juice from Ann Louise Gittleman, a health pioneer and detox expert. In her book *The Fat Flush Plan* she explains that cranberry juice cleanses the lymphatic system, responsible for carrying toxins away from the cells and body tissues, which can help eliminate stubborn fat. Cranberry juice is rich in phytonutrients (anthocyanins, catechins, luteins, and quercetin), which help to keep your liver's detoxification pathways open, so they aren't jammed up by environmental pollutants, trans fats, sugars, and other toxins. In other words, cranberry juice helps "take out the trash."

Steps 4, 5, and 6: Lunch, Dinner, and Bedtime Snack

The nutritional components of lunch and dinner are based on what your body needs most at midday and in the evening to help you perform at your peak. Both meals include protein, as it is vital for complete detoxification. Remember, I suggest *minimal* requirements of protein for each of these meals and *no maximum*. Why is protein so important? The liver uses amino acids such as glycine and cysteine to transport toxins out of the body. These amino acids are found in protein. I do not like juice or fasting cleanses, because they deprive the body of these amino acids. The body prepares toxins for removal, but when the amino acids needed to transport them never show up, the liver is forced to reprocess and store these toxins once again. Do not be afraid of protein; it's essential to complete detoxification.

In addition to protein, lunch includes good fats and vegetables to stabilize blood sugar, enhancing fat loss and keeping stress hormones at bay. This combination also enhances brain function by stimulating dopamine and acetylcholine, brain neurotransmitters that enhance drive, focus, and memory. At dinnertime, it's time to calm your body down and prepare it for good sleep. I've introduced carbs at dinner to enhance this process.

Don't freak! Remember, eating carbs at night *will not make you fat.* But they will help you get a good night's sleep. Carbs stimulate the brain to produce serotonin, a chemical that promotes relaxation and sleep. This means you can kiss your Xanax, Ambien, or Sleep-Eze good-bye once and for all; you no longer need them and you will be eliminating another toxin that's putting stress on your body.

You will cap the night off with a snack that includes a protein containing the amino acid tryptophan, the precursor to serotonin. This snack replicates post–Thanksgiving dinner drowsiness. The benefit? A better night's sleep. When was the last time you had one of those?

Phase 1: 7-Day Sample Meal Plan

Below is a sample 7-day meal plan for the Reset. As you'll see, meals can be supersimple and basic or, if you're a foodie, you can really dial up some fantastic dishes. As long as you stick with the approved foods and the nutritional requirements for each meal, you can get as creative as you like. My wife loves trying out new dishes during our Reset periods. I've included a few of our favorites in the meal plan. You'll find the recipes in Chapter 12.

Pay attention to the servings of fats, carbs, and fruits in each recipe and adjust as needed to fit your requirements. Remember, you can eat as much protein and vegetables as you want.

			PHASE 1 SAMPLE MEAL PLAN			
	Breakfast	Morning Snack	Lunch	Afternoon Snack	Dinner	Bedtime
Day 1	Detox Smoothie: The CEO	Cranberry Juice Cocktail	Fajita Bowl with Pico de Gallo	Green Tea	Yam, Chicken, and Kale Stir-Fry	Pineapple Cottage Cheese
Day 2	Detox Smoothie: Mr. Clean	Cranberry Juice Cocktail	Asian Meatballs Raw Kale and Brussels Sprout Salad	Green Tea	Moussaka	Mango Pecans
Day 3	Detox Smoothie: Hello Mojo	Cranberry Juice Cocktail	Shredded Pork Lettuce Wraps with Avocado Dressing	Green Tea	Hearty Bison Stew	Blackberries Cashews
Day 4	Detox Smoothie: The Energizer Bunny	Cranberry Juice Cocktail	Kabobs with Chimichurri Sauce Salad with Greek Vinaigrette Dressing	Green Tea	Halibut Tacos with Jicama Shells and Cilantro Slaw	Cherries Cottage Cheese
Day 5	Detox Smoothie: Gut Be Gone	Cranberry Juice Cocktail	Mini Meatloaf Roasted Vegetables	Green Tea	Fajita Bowl with Pico de Gallo Kicked-Up Quinoa Salad	Pineapple Cashews
Day 6	Detox Smoothie: The Graduate	Cranberry Juice Cocktail	Ground Chicken Lettuce Wraps Creamed Veggie Soup	Green Tea	Kabobs with Chimichurri Sauce Smashed and Fried Red Potatoes	Orange Slices Pecans
Day 7	Detox Smoothie: Chillaxin'	Cranberry Juice Cocktail	Sea Bass with Garlic, Ginger, and Coconut Oil Roasted Vegetables	Green Tea	Turkey Sliders with Pickled Red Onions Yam or Sweet Potato Fries	Plum Cottage Cheese

12

The Stark Naked 21-Day Metabolic Reset Recipes

Breakfast

All of the following smoothies are approved for use during the Stark Naked 21-Day Metabolic Reset. Each smoothie supports the foundational needs required at breakfast for you to succeed on this program. If you would like extra support in a specific area, try the smoothie targeted to your needs.

Also, if a cold smoothie upsets your stomach or causes diarrhea, try drinking a room-temperature smoothie instead.

Each recipe makes one smoothie, unless otherwise noted.

Note: If you have been diagnosed with gout or hypothyroidism, use the Safe Detox Smoothie (p. 228) during the Reset. With these conditions, you need to limit the amount of cruciferous greens you consume and should eat kale, spinach, and Swiss chard only once in a while. You also have the option of replacing kale, spinach, and chard with romaine lettuce in the other smoothies.

The Beginner

(A Safe Place to Start)

If you are new to green smoothies, this is the safest place to start. My clients consistently rank this as one of their favorites.

1 handful kale
1 handful spinach
1 cup papaya or mango
1 green apple with peel, seeded, cored, and chopped
2 tablespoons heavy whipping cream
1 cup water

Blend ingredients until smooth, adding more water and/or ice to reach the desired consistency.

The CEO

(Enhanced Brain Performance)

Life as a CEO requires high cognitive ability to be successful. Stress can negatively affect brain function, leading to foggy thinking, reduced memory, poor judgment, and reduced capacity to learn. Packed with powerful brain-enhancing ingredients, this smoothie is for you if you feel you need a CEO-level boost of brain power.

2 handfuls spinach
2 celery stalks
½ cup mixed berries (no blueberries)
½ cup unsweetened canned coconut milk
1 tablespoon coconut oil
6 ounces yerba mate tea
Optional: 1 sprig fresh rosemary, leaves removed and
    finely chopped

Blend ingredients until smooth, adding water and/or ice to reach the desired consistency.

The Energizer Bunny

(Energy Boost)

If you have a tough time finding the energy to get going in the mornings, then this smoothie is for you. These ingredients will wake you up, get you moving, and keep you going until lunch with stable, long-lasting energy.

1 handful kale
1 handful spinach
¼ avocado
½ cup pineapple
1 cup unsweetened canned coconut milk
6 ounces room-temperature green tea
1 teaspoon cinnamon
Optional: 1 teaspoon maca powder

Blend ingredients until smooth, adding water and/or ice to reach the desired consistency.

Mama's Little Helper

(Calm, Cool, and Collected)

I remember being a young trainer and listening to mothers talk about their "mama's little helpers." When I asked what that meant, they laughed and told me it was what they used to keep stress and anxiety at bay, such as Xanax. This anti-anxiety smoothie is a great, natural "mama's little helper." Built to fight high stress and anxiety, it is guaranteed to keep you calm, cool, and collected.

2 handfuls kale
½ cup diced mango
½ cup diced peaches
1 cup unsweetened almond milk

¼ **cup mint**
1 **teaspoon chia seeds**
1 **tablespoon cocoa powder**

Blend ingredients until smooth, adding water and/or ice to reach the desired consistency.

Mr. Clean

(Loving Your Liver)

If you struggle with waking between 1:00 and 3:00 A.M. most nights or you have horrible morning energy, this is the smoothie for you. Your liver needs extra support, and this smoothie is packed with known natural liver aids that help detoxification. It will improve your quality of sleep and boost your morning energy.

2 handfuls kale
½ **cup pineapple**
½ **cup mango**
1 **cup unsweetened canned coconut milk**
2–3 dandelion leaves
¼ **teaspoon ground turmeric**

Blend ingredients until smooth, adding water and/or ice to reach the desired consistency.

Hello Mojo

(The Power to Shag)

If your mojo is so low you would rather sleep than shag, this is the smoothie for you. A natural aphrodisiac in a glass for both men and women, it is packed full of natural ingredients to boost sex drive and enhance blood flow. Life's more fun when it's flowing with mojo! Warning: only drink if you desire more action in the bedroom.

1 handful spinach
1 handful Swiss chard
2 celery stalks
½ avocado
½ cup blackberries or strawberries
½ cup chopped watermelon
1 tablespoon maca powder
1 teaspoon cinnamon

Blend ingredients until smooth, adding water and/or ice to reach the desired consistency.

Svelte

(A Gracefully Slender Figure)

This smoothie is great if you're looking for added fat-burning capabilities to enhance your figure. Packed full of foods that contain known fat-burning nutrients, this smoothie will add extra firepower to attack your waistline.

2 handfuls spinach
1 small cucumber, chopped
1 green apple with peel, seeded, cored, and chopped
1 cup unsweetened canned coconut milk
6 ounces green tea, chilled
1 teaspoon cinnamon
Optional: 1 jalapeño, stem removed

Blend ingredients until smooth, adding water and/or ice to reach the desired consistency.

Gut Be Gone

(Better Digestion)

If you suffer from digestive problems like bloating, gas, and acid reflux, this is the smoothie for you. Packed full of gut aids, this smoothie replenishes good gut bacteria and digestive enzymes and reduces gut inflammation.

2 handfuls spinach
½ avocado
1 cup pineapple
1 cup unsweetened canned coconut milk
½-inch slice fresh ginger
1 tablespoon chia seeds
Optional: 1 serving probiotic powder

Blend ingredients until smooth, adding water and/or ice to reach the desired consistency.

Chillaxin'

(A Little Chillin' Plus a Little Relaxin')

If you live a highly driven life that's full of stress, then this is the smoothie for you. Packed full of foods that naturally fight stress, this smoothie will offset the damage a high-stress day causes your body. Chillaxin' at breakfast is a great way to start the day.

1 handful spinach
1 handful Swiss chard
½ avocado
1 cup blackberries
1 cup unsweetened almond milk
1 tablespoon cocoa powder
Optional: 1 serving probiotic powder

Blend ingredients until smooth, adding water and/or ice to reach the desired consistency.

Pretty Hot and Tempting

(Some Like It Hot!)

Want a little spice in your life? This smoothie turns up the heat, enhancing blood flow, reducing inflammation, and helping to burn stubborn belly fat.

2 handfuls kale
½ cucumber, chopped
1 bell pepper, cored and chopped
1 cup mango
1 cup unsweetened canned coconut milk
½-inch piece of jalapeño (remove seeds to reduce heat)
Optional: ½-inch slice fresh ginger

Blend ingredients until smooth, adding water and/or ice to reach the desired consistency.

The Graduate

(Love Me Some Veggies)

If you love veggies, you'll love this smoothie, but be warned: it tastes supergreen. It's crazy healthy, but this smoothie is definitely for the advanced green-smoothie drinker.

1 handful kale
1 handful spinach
2 celery stalks, chopped
1 small cucumber, chopped
1 apple with peel, seeded, cored, and chopped

1 cup unsweetened almond milk
½ lime, peeled

Blend ingredients until smooth, adding water and/or ice to reach the desired consistency.

Headache No More

(Stop the Pounding)

In the first 3 to 5 days of the Reset you may experience headaches, especially if you're coming off coffee. It's normal and only lasts a few days, but this smoothie is a blessing.

2 handfuls spinach
1 small cucumber
1 apple with peel, seeded, cored, and chopped
½ cup pineapple
1 cup unsweetened canned coconut milk
1 teaspoon cinnamon
½-inch slice fresh ginger

Blend ingredients until smooth, adding water and/or ice to reach the desired consistency.

Safe Detox Smoothie

(Good for Gout and Hypothyroidism)

If you have been diagnosed with gout or hypothyroidism, this is the only smoothie you should use during the Reset, as you need to limit the amount of cruciferous greens you consume. Romaine lettuce is a safe choice.

2 handfuls romaine lettuce
½ cup parsley

¼ **cucumber**

½ **cup mango or pineapple chunks**

6 ounces water

1 tablespoon coconut oil

Blend ingredients until smooth, adding water and/or ice to reach the desired consistency.

Lunch and Dinner

When my clients go on the Stark Naked 21-Day Metabolic Reset, their biggest worry is whether they can stick with the eating plan. No matter how many times I tell them it's easier than they think to eat the right foods for their body, they still panic.

Although I am a master at the grill, I will admit I am no chef in the kitchen. My criteria for every recipe in this book was that it had to be so easy to follow, prepare, and cook that even a klutz in the kitchen like me could make it!

Since I am not a master in the kitchen, I decided to ask my friend and chef extraordinaire Rebecca Clubb, owner of Whole Health Everyday, to step in. Based on my guidelines, Rebecca provided these amazing and delicious recipes to use throughout your 21-day reset and beyond.

Rebecca is the private chef for many of my clients here at Stark and a favorite chef of many of our professional athletes. Not only is Rebecca an incredibly talented chef; she is also someone who suffered from many common food sensitivities. She understands how hard it can be to remove typical food triggers, while still finding a way to keep your nutrition choices interesting and enjoyable. As a result of her own struggles, she has now committed her life to providing safe and incredible healthy meals for people with food sensitivities without having to cut the flavor and comfort we all crave from our food.

Serving sizes for protein, vegetables, fat, carbs, and fruit are listed for each recipe, except where the amount included does not equal one complete serving. Pay particular attention to the amounts of fats, carbs, and fruits and adjust as needed to stay within your serving requirements. There is no limit to the amounts of protein and vegetables you can eat during the Reset. We've designed these recipes to be very flexible and forgiving if you need to dial back the fat or carbs.

Note: For chicken and vegetable broth, choose organic, if possible, and brands that do not add sugar, corn syrup, or thickeners such as wheat.

Bon appetit!

Lunch and Dinner Protein-Based Mains

Bison Meatballs with San Marzano Sauce

2 servings of protein
2½ servings of fat (2 in meatballs and ½ in 1 cup sauce)

For the meatballs
  2 tablespoons extra virgin olive oil
  3 tablespoons finely diced onion
  1 clove garlic, minced
  6 ounces ground bison
  1 tablespoon finely chopped parsley
  Salt and pepper, to taste

For the sauce
  2 tablespoons extra virgin olive oil
  1 small onion, roughly chopped
  3 cloves garlic, chopped
  1 28-ounce can organic San Marzano tomatoes
  ¼ cup chiffonade fresh basil
  Salt and pepper, to taste

Preheat the oven to 350°F.

To make the meatballs: Heat the oil in a small sauté pan and add the onions. Sauté over medium-low heat until the onions caramelize. Add the garlic and continue to cook for another minute. Remove from the heat.

In a large bowl, combine the onions (with all the oil from the pan) with the ground bison and parsley. Season with salt and pepper.

Form a small amount of the mixture into a test patty and cook in the sauté pan. Adjust seasonings to taste.

Form the remaining mixture into 4 small balls. Place the meatballs on a parchment-lined baking sheet and bake 15 minutes.

To make the sauce: Heat the oil in a small sauce pot and sauté the onion and garlic until just opaque. Add the basil and continue to cook for 1 minute. Add the tomatoes and stir. Let simmer for 30 minutes, then blend with an immersion blender or in a conventional blender until the desired consistency and return the mixture to the pot. Add salt and pepper to taste.

To serve: Serve meatballs with 1 cup of sauce. Freeze the remaining sauce in 1-cup portions for later use.

Turkey Sliders with Pickled Red Onions

2 servings of protein
2 servings of fat

½ red onion, thinly sliced
Red wine vinegar
2 drops stevia
2 tablespoons extra virgin olive oil
¼ cup finely chopped onion
1 garlic clove, finely chopped
6 ounces ground turkey
1 teaspoon dried marjoram

2 pinches salt, divided
Pinch of white pepper
4 lettuce leaves
2 slices tomato

Place the red onion slices in a small bowl and cover with red wine vinegar. Stir in 2 drops stevia and a pinch of salt. Let sit for at least 30 minutes.

Heat the oil in a sauté pan and sauté the onions until they are a light caramel color. Add the garlic and cook another minute. Remove from the heat.

In a bowl, combine the onions (with all the oil from the pan), turkey, marjoram, a pinch of salt, and a pinch of white pepper.

Place the sauté pan over medium heat. Form a small amount of the turkey mixture into a small test patty and cook on each side until the turkey is cooked through (white with no pink). Taste and adjust seasoning.

Form the meat into 2 small patties and cook in the sauté pan for about 2 to 3 minutes on each side, until lightly browned and cooked through.

Serve the patties on the lettuce leaves topped with pickled red onions and tomato slices.

Ground Chicken Lettuce Wraps

2 servings of protein
4 servings of vegetables
1 serving of fat

1 tablespoon sesame oil
1 garlic clove, roughly chopped
1 tablespoon roughly chopped ginger
2 green onions, sliced, white and green parts separated

6 ounces ground chicken

4 cups finely chopped water chestnuts

1–2 tablespoons coconut aminos (great alternative to soy sauce)

Pepper, to taste

4 butter lettuce leaves

Cilantro leaves, for garnish

Heat the sesame oil in a sauté pan and add the garlic, ginger, and white part of the green onions. After the garlic and ginger become fragrant, add the ground chicken. Make sure to break up the chicken and cook until lightly browned. Add the water chestnuts and season with coconut aminos, pepper, and additional sesame oil to taste.

Spoon the mixture into the centers of the four lettuce leaves, dividing evenly, and garnish with cilantro and green onions.

Fajita Bowl with Pico de Gallo

2 servings of protein

2 servings of vegetables

2 servings of fat

For the fajita bowl

6 ounces chicken, bison, or buffalo, sliced into strips

Salt and pepper, to taste

Cumin, to taste

Chipotle pepper, to taste (optional)

2 tablespoons coconut oil, extra virgin olive oil, or ghee, divided

1 onion (any kind), sliced into thin strips

1 clove garlic, chopped

1½ cups thinly sliced bell pepper, any color

½ jalapeño, seeded and sliced into thin strips

Paprika, to taste

For the pico de gallo
   1 Roma tomato, chopped
   1 tablespoon finely chopped onion
   1 clove garlic, chopped
   ½ jalapeño, seeded and chopped
   Juice of ½ lime
   Salt and pepper, to taste

Sprinkle the strips of meat with salt, pepper, cumin, and chipotle pepper.

Heat 1 tablespoon coconut oil in a sauté pan and add the meat. Let the meat sear until it is browned and crisp on one side, then flip and sear the other side. Remove the meat from the pan and place in a large bowl.

Add the remaining oil and onions to the pan and sauté until they become golden brown. Add the garlic, peppers, and jalapeños. Once the peppers are nearly cooked through, season with salt, pepper, cumin, chipotle, and paprika to taste. Sauté until the peppers are cooked through. Remove to the bowl with the meat and toss.

To make the pico de gallo: In a small bowl combine all the ingredients. Season to taste.

To serve: Top the meat and peppers with pico de gallo.

Kabobs with Chimichurri Sauce

2 servings of protein
2 servings of vegetables
2 servings of fat (in ¼ cup sauce)

For the kabobs
   6 ounces chicken, buffalo, or bison, cut into 1-inch cubes
   2 cups veggies, such as mushrooms, zucchini, bell peppers,
      or onions, cut into 1-inch cubes

**Skewers, wooden or metal (if using wooden skewers and grilling
the kabobs over an open flame, soak them in water for at least an
hour before using)**

For the chimichurri sauce
½ cup extra virgin olive oil
¼ bunch (½ cup) fresh Italian parsley, most of the stems removed
1 bunch (2 cups) fresh cilantro, most of the stems removed
1 tablespoon fresh oregano or 2 teaspoons dried
2–4 garlic cloves, peeled
2 tablespoons chopped red onion
2–3 tablespoons red wine vinegar
½ teaspoon ground cumin
Pinch of red pepper flakes (optional)
Sea salt and white pepper, to taste

Place the meat and vegetables on skewers, alternating meat and
vegetables or making separate meat and vegetable skewers.

To make the sauce: In a food processor or blender, add ¼ cup of
olive oil and the rest of the ingredients. Blend until well combined.
Slowly add the remaining oil until at the desired consistency. Taste
for seasoning and adjust salt, cumin, vinegar, and pepper as desired.

Coat the skewered meat and veggies with 1 tablespoon of the
sauce and let marinate at least 30 minutes or overnight. Set aside
3 tablespoons for serving, and reserve the remaining ¾ cup sauce
for another use.

Skewers may be grilled on an outdoor grill, in a grill pan, or
seared in a sauté pan. Grill over medium-high heat until browned
on all sides and cooked through.

Mini Meatloaf

2 servings of protein
2 servings of fat

2 tablespoons extra virgin olive oil
3 tablespoons finely diced onion (any kind)
1 clove garlic, minced
6 ounces ground bison
1 tablespoon finely chopped parsley
Salt and white pepper, to taste
1 Roma tomato, chopped
2 leaves of fresh basil, chopped
Pinch of red pepper flakes

Preheat the oven to 350°F.

Heat the oil in a small sauté pan over medium-low heat and add the onion. Sauté until the onion caramelizes. Add the garlic and continue to cook for another minute. Remove from the heat.

In a bowl, combine the onions (with all the oil from the pan), bison, parsley, a pinch of salt, and a pinch of white pepper.

Place the sauté pan over medium-low heat. Form a small amount of the bison mixture into a small test patty and cook on each side until the meat is cooked through. Taste and adjust seasoning as desired.

On a parchment-lined baking sheet, form the bison mixture into a loaf shape with a well down the middle.

In a small bowl, combine the tomato, basil, red pepper flakes, salt, and pepper and spoon the mixture into the well. Bake the meatloaf for 25 minutes. Slice and serve.

Shredded Pork Lettuce Wraps

2 servings of protein

6 ounces pork loin, cut into 1-inch pieces
1 garlic clove, roughly chopped
1 tablespoon roughly chopped ginger
2 tablespoons coconut aminos (great alternative to soy sauce)
1 star anise
4 drops stevia
½ cup vegetable broth
¼ teaspoon pepper
4 romaine lettuce leaves
2 green onions, sliced
Bean sprouts, for garnish
Cilantro leaves, for garnish
Sriracha sauce, for garnish
1 lime wedge

In a small sauce pot, combine the pork, garlic, ginger, coconut aminos, star anise, stevia, vegetable broth, and pepper. Cover and simmer over low heat about 30 minutes or until the meat is cooked through. Shred the pork. Strain and discard the excess liquid.

Serve the shredded pork on the lettuce leaves and garnish with green onions, bean sprouts, cilantro, and sriracha. Squeeze lime over the top.

Sea Bass with Garlic, Ginger, and Coconut Oil

2 servings of protein
1 serving of fat

Zest of ½ lemon
1 clove garlic, minced

1 teaspoon grated ginger

1 tablespoon coconut oil, divided

6 ounces wild sea bass

Salt and white pepper, to taste

Lemon wedges, for serving

Preheat the oven to 400°F.

In a small bowl, combine the lemon zest, garlic, ginger, and 1½ teaspoons coconut oil. Rub the mixture onto the top of the sea bass. Let sit in refrigerator for 30 minutes to 2 hours.

Season sea bass with salt and pepper.

Heat a nonstick sauté pan over medium-high heat and add remaining 1½ teaspoons coconut oil. When the oil is hot, place the sea bass face down (presentation side), skin side up. Let the fish sear without disturbing it for about 2 minutes. When it is a little more than golden brown, flip the sea bass over and sear for another 2 minutes.

To finish cooking the fish, place the pan in the oven for 2 to 4 minutes or until the thickest part of the fish flakes easily.

Remove from the oven and let sit 5 minutes before serving. Serve with lemon wedges.

Asian Meatballs

5+ servings of protein

2 servings of fat

1 pound ground turkey

2 tablespoons ground flax mixed with 4 tablespoons water (let sit for 5 minutes)

1½ tablespoons minced ginger

¼ teaspoon white pepper

½ cup finely chopped cilantro

4 green onions, white and green parts, finely chopped
1½ tablespoons coconut aminos or soy sauce
1 tablespoon sesame oil
1 teaspoon toasted sesame oil

Preheat the oven to 400°F.
In a large bowl, combine all the ingredients.
Form the mixture into 16 balls and place on a parchment-lined baking sheet. Bake for 25 minutes.

Dinner-Only Protein-Based Mains
(Containing Approved Complex Carbs)

Halibut Tacos with Jicama Shells and Cilantro Slaw

2 servings of protein
2 servings of fat
1 serving of carbohydrates (or more, depending on the size of jicama)

This recipe can be adjusted in many ways for your own tastes by using ground or sliced meat instead of fish. You can use any meat on the approved-foods list such as duck, chicken, bison, or even turkey! To create jicama taco shells, you will need a basic mandolin slicer.

1 jicama
1 lime, zested and juiced
1 clove garlic, finely chopped
½ teaspoon ground cumin
½ bunch cilantro, stems removed and finely chopped (reserve some for garnish, if desired)
2 green onions, green and white parts, finely chopped
1 tablespoon extra virgin olive oil or avocado oil
Sea salt and white pepper, to taste

6 ounces wild halibut

½ cup thinly sliced or shredded savoy cabbage

1 tablespoon coconut oil

1 Roma tomato, diced and sprinkled with sea salt and black pepper

1 teaspoon finely diced jalapeño

Use a sharp knife to cut off one end of the jicama and then, working around the bulb, cut off the rough skin. Use a knife or vegetable peeler to make a smooth surface around the jicama. Slice the jicama on a mandolin into thin rounds. The slices should look like taco shells.

Combine the lime zest, juice, garlic, cumin, cilantro, greens onions, olive or avocado oil, salt, and pepper in a medium-size bowl, mashing with the back of a fork. Coat the halibut with 1 tablespoon of the sauce and let it marinate for 10 to 15 minutes.

Toss the remaining sauce with the cabbage, adjusting seasoning to taste.

Heat the coconut oil in a small nonstick sauté pan over medium-high heat. Cook the halibut until the fish is just opaque and flakes easily with a fork, about 2 to 3 minutes per side. Transfer the fish to a plate and cut into pieces.

Serve the fish inside jicama taco shells with slaw, tomato, and jalapeño. Garnish with extra cilantro.

Hearty Bison Stew

2 servings of protein

2 servings of fat

3 servings of carbohydrates

6 ounces bison, cubed

2 tablespoons organic butter, ghee, or extra virgin olive oil

1 yellow onion, roughly chopped

2 garlic cloves, roughly chopped
2 cups vegetable broth
1 cup peeled and cubed parsnip
1 cup peeled and cubed yam or sweet potato
1 cup peeled and cubed rutabaga
Salt and white pepper, to taste
1 bay leaf
Pinch of thyme

Sprinkle the bison cubes with a little salt and pepper.

Heat the butter, ghee, or oil in a medium saucepan. Add the bison cubes, and sear them on all sides. Remove them to a small bowl.

Add the onions to the same saucepan used to cook the bison and sauté over medium heat, stirring often until they start to caramelize and become slightly browned. Add the garlic and continue to cook for another minute.

Add the broth, the rest of the ingredients, and the bison. Bring to a simmer, then lower heat, and cook for about 1 hour or until veggies are tender. The length of time will depend on the size of vegetables.

Remove the bay leaf. Adjust salt, pepper, and thyme to taste.

Moussaka

5+ servings of protein
15 servings of vegetables
6 servings of fat
1 serving of carbohydrates

1 large eggplant (about 2 pounds), peeled and cut into 1-inch cubes (choose one that is heavy for its size)
6 tablespoons extra virgin olive oil, divided
3 cups vegetable or chicken broth

1 medium red potato, cut unto 1-inch pieces

1 head cauliflower, cored and cut into florets

2 yellow onions, chopped

4 garlic cloves, chopped

1 pound ground lamb, bison, or turkey

1 28-ounce can San Marzano tomatoes, drained and crushed

1 tablespoon tomato paste

½ cup chopped parsley

2 teaspoons dried (or 1 tablespoon fresh) oregano

1 teaspoon cinnamon

Salt and white pepper, to taste

Preheat the oven to 400°F.

Sprinkle the eggplant cubes with a little salt and set them aside in a strainer to drain for about 30 minutes. Once they have let go of some moisture, toss them with 4 tablespoons of olive oil and pepper. Bake them in a 9 x 13-inch baking dish for 20 to 30 minutes or until golden. Remove from the oven.

Heat the broth in a small saucepan over medium heat and add the potato and cauliflower. Simmer over medium heat until they are soft, but not mushy. Remove the potato and cauliflower pieces to a blender or food processor and whip until they reach the consistency of mashed potatoes. Add some of the broth from the pot as needed to get to the desired consistency. Taste for seasoning and add salt and pepper if needed.

In a large sauté pan add the remaining 2 tablespoons oil and onions. Sauté the onions over medium heat, stirring often, until they become slightly browned. Add the garlic and continue to cook for another minute. Add the ground meat and continue to cook, breaking up the meat, until cooked through. Stir in the tomatoes, tomato paste, parsley, oregano, and cinnamon. Taste for seasoning and add salt and pepper to taste.

Spread the meat mixture over the eggplant. Top with whipped cauliflower, spreading evenly over the meat.

Broil 3 to 5 minutes, or until the top is browned.

Yam, Chicken, and Kale Stir-Fry

2 servings of protein
2 servings of vegetables
3 servings of fat
1 serving of carbohydrates

6 ounces chicken breast
1 tablespoon extra virgin olive oil
1 cup cubed sweet potato or yam
2 tablespoons coconut oil
1 tablespoon finely chopped garlic
1 tablespoon finely chopped ginger
1 tablespoon turmeric
2 cups thinly sliced and destemmed kale
Salt and pepper, to taste

Preheat the oven to 400°F. Line a baking sheet with parchment paper.

Place the chicken breast on the sheet. Drizzle with olive oil and sprinkle with salt and pepper. Add the cubed sweet potato or yam on the sheet pan.

Bake for 30 minutes or until the chicken is cooked through and juices run clear. Cool and shred chicken. Once the yam is soft, remove it. It may take only 20 minutes.

Heat the coconut oil in a wok or sauté pan over medium heat. Add garlic and ginger and sauté for just a minute or two, then add the yams, chicken, and turmeric. Once the kale is wilted, season with salt and pepper to taste.

Creamed Veggie Soup

4 servings of vegetables
1 serving of fat

Make this a complete meal by adding protein such as baked, cubed, or shredded chicken.

1 tablespoon extra virgin olive oil, coconut oil, or ghee
½ yellow or white onion, chopped
1 clove garlic, chopped
4 cups chopped asparagus, cauliflower, or other approved
    vegetable of your choice
4 cups vegetable broth
Salt and pepper, to taste

In a medium-size pot, heat the oil over medium heat and sauté the onion and garlic until tender. Add the vegetables and broth and bring to a boil. Lower the heat to a simmer and cook until vegetables are tender.

Remove the vegetables to a blender with just enough of the broth to help it blend. Puree the vegetables until they reach the desired consistency, adding more broth as needed. Taste for seasoning, and add salt and pepper as desired.

Raw Kale and Brussels Sprout Salad

2 servings of vegetables
2 servings of fat (in 3 tablespoons of dressing)

For the salad
    1½ cups destemmed kale, cut into thin strips
    ½ cup thinly sliced Brussels sprouts

For the dressing
¼ cup lemon juice
1 tablespoon Dijon mustard
1 tablespoon finely chopped shallot
½ cup extra virgin olive oil
Salt and pepper, to taste
Fresh thyme leaves, to taste
Chives, to taste
Lemon zest, to taste

Combine all dressing ingredients in a jar with tight-fitting lid and shake. Taste. Adjust seasoning to your taste.

Toss kale and Brussels sprouts with 3 tablespoons of dressing. Reserve remaining dressing for another use.

Serve topped with chives, thyme, and lemon zest.

Roasted Vegetables

Varies

Need to add more vegetables to a meal? It's easy to makes as many servings as you need by roasting them. The potential flavor combinations are endless!

The fat content will depend on how much oil you add to the vegetables before roasting. A little goes a long way!

Extra virgin olive oil (about 1 tablespoon per 2 cups of vegetables)
Sea salt and white pepper, to taste

Any combination of these vegetables
Acorn squash, peeled, seeded, and cut into 1-inch wedges
Butternut squash, peeled, seeded, and cut into 1-inch pieces
Parsnips, peeled, and cut into 1-inch pieces
Brussels sprouts, halved
Asparagus, rough ends cut off

Green beans, ends trimmed

Cabbage, cut into 1-inch rounds

Cauliflower, cut into florets

Accents to add for additional flavor

Garlic	Chives	Lime zest
Rosemary	Balsamic vinegar	Curry powder
Sage	Dijon mustard	Paprika
Thyme	Sesame oil	Cumin
Tarragon	Soy sauce	Cinnamon
Mint	Lemon zest	Nutmeg
Parsley	Orange zest	

Suggested accent matchings

Acorn squash: cinnamon, sage, or nutmeg

Butternut squash: sage

Parsnips: curry powder, lemon, nutmeg, or tarragon

Brussels sprouts: drizzle with balsamic vinegar when they come out
    of the oven and top with rosemary, Dijon mustard, or thyme

Asparagus: garlic, lime, mint, balsamic vinegar, or orange zest

Green beans: soy sauce, sesame oil, or garlic

Cabbage: paprika, parsley, or garlic

Cauliflower: chives, parsley, curry powder, or lemon zest

Preheat the oven to 450°F. Line a baking sheet with parchment paper.

In a large bowl, toss the vegetables with extra virgin olive oil, sea salt, and white pepper until coated. Add accents for more flavor.

Spread the vegetables on the baking sheet. Make sure veggies are in a single layer and not piled up, which will result in steaming them rather than roasting.

Roast green beans and asparagus about 15 minutes and other veggies up to 45 minutes. Toss and stir the veggies halfway through anticipated cooking time. When the veggies are browned, they are done! Be careful not to char them.

Complex Carbohydrate Sides

Coconut-Ginger Rice

8+ servings of fat
2 servings of carbohydrates

1 cup jasmine rice
1 teaspoon coconut oil
3 tablespoons diced shallots
2 teaspoons minced ginger
½ cup unsweetened canned coconut milk
1 cup vegetable broth
¼ teaspoon salt
2 tablespoons chopped chives
Zest of 1 lime

Rinse the rice in cool water.

Heat the oil in a small pot over medium heat. Add the shallots and sauté for about 2 minutes. Add the ginger and continue to cook about 1 more minute. Add the rice and continue to stir for another 2 minutes until the rice gives off a nutty aroma.

Add the coconut milk, broth, and salt and bring to a simmer. Reduce the heat to low, cover, and simmer until all the liquid is absorbed, about 15 minutes.

Toss the rice with chives and serve topped with lime zest.

Kicked-Up Quinoa Salad

6 servings of vegetables
3 servings of carbohydrates
2 servings of fat

1 cup quinoa
2 cups water or chicken or vegetable broth

4 green onions, white and green parts, sliced

2 tablespoons diced white onion

1 jalapeño, finely diced

1 cup cherry tomatoes, quartered

1 yellow bell pepper, diced

½ bunch cilantro, stems removed and finely chopped (about ½ cup)

1 avocado, diced (about 1 cup)

Zest and juice of 1 lime

1 tablespoon adobo sauce or to taste

Sea salt and black pepper, to taste

4 cups spinach, roughly chopped

Rinse the quinoa under cool water.

Bring the water or broth to a boil, add the quinoa, reduce the heat, and cover. Let simmer until all the broth is absorbed, about 11 minutes. Remove from the heat. Remove the cover, lay a few paper towels over the pot, and place the cover back on. Let this sit for another 5 minutes. Remove the cover and towels, fluff with a fork, and let cool. If you want it to cool quickly, you can spread it out on a sheet pan.

Toss cooled quinoa with remaining ingredients, green onions through salt and pepper. Adjust seasoning to taste. Serve over spinach.

Smashed and Fried Red Potatoes

2 servings of fat
2 servings of carbohydrates

1 pound (7–9) red potatoes

1 teaspoon salt, plus more to taste

Pepper, to taste

Garlic powder, to taste
2 tablespoons extra virgin olive oil, ghee, or coconut oil
2 tablespoons chopped parsley

Wash the potatoes and add to a pot with 1 teaspoon of salt and enough water to cover. Bring to a boil and simmer until the potatoes are tender, about 20 minutes. Remove the potatoes and let cool.

With the back of a spatula press down on each potato and flatten it. Sprinkle with salt, pepper, and garlic powder.

Heat the oil or ghee in a pan and fry each potato until golden brown. Flip and brown the other side. Remove and serve topped with parsley.

Yam or Sweet Potato Fries

3 servings of fat
6 servings of carbohydrates (depending on the size of the potatoes or yams)

3 medium sweet potatoes or yams
3 tablespoons extra virgin olive oil
Sea salt and white or black pepper, to taste
Garlic powder (optional)
Paprika (optional)

Preheat the oven to 450°F. Line a baking sheet with parchment paper.

Wash and peel the sweet potatoes or yams. Cut them into thick steak fries or ¼-inch thick strips.

In a bowl, toss the potatoes with extra virgin olive oil and sprinkle with sea salt and white or black pepper. Sprinkle with garlic powder and paprika, if using. Toss until coated.

Spread the potatoes on baking sheet. Make sure the fries are in a single layer and not piled up, which will result in steaming rather than roasting them. Roast for 20 to 40 minutes, tossing occasionally, until golden brown. Roasting time depends on the size and thickness of the fries.

Salad Dressings

Greek Vinaigrette Dressing

8–12 servings of fat

¼ cup red wine vinegar
½ teaspoon salt
¼ teaspoon white pepper
½ teaspoon dried oregano
¼ teaspoon dried mint
½–¾ cup extra virgin olive oil

In a small bowl whisk the vinegar and salt. Add the pepper, oregano, and mint. Slowly drizzle in ½ cup of olive oil while continuing to whisk. Taste and add more olive oil and seasonings as desired. You may also combine all ingredients in a tightly sealed jar and shake vigorously to emulsify.

Avocado Dressing

4 servings of fat

Juice of 1 lemon or lime, divided
2 tablespoons water
1 ripe avocado, flesh removed
2 tablespoons avocado oil or olive oil

1 small clove garlic
½ cup cilantro leaves
Salt and white pepper, to taste
Stevia (optional)

In a blender or food processor, combine 1 tablespoon of the lemon juice with the rest of the ingredients (start with a pinch of salt and pepper). Blend until smooth. Taste and add more lemon juice and adjust seasoning as desired. Thin with additional water as needed to reach a dressing consistency. If using stevia to sweeten, start with one drop and taste before adding more.

▶ PART FIVE

YOU'VE RESET, NOW OPTIMIZE

13

Phase 2

The Stark Naked High-Performance Optimized Nutrition Plan

CONGRATULATIONS!

Now that you have completed Phase 1, the Stark Naked 21-Day Metabolic Reset, and healed your metabolism, it's time to optimize it with Phase 2, the Stark Naked High-Performance Optimized Nutrition Plan.

During the past three weeks, your metabolism has recovered from all of the damage your stress has caused. You feel great, don't you? You should be able to look in the mirror and say, "I don't ever remember *feeling* or *looking* this good!" Let's keep it that way!

The Stark Naked High-Performance Optimized Nutrition Plan is an easy way to sustain a long-term program that provides you with our exclusive nutritional strategies, which are currently being used only with a small population of really healthy and truly resilient high achievers in the world. These strategies create a resiliency to high levels of stress, protecting the body from falling back into the Metabolic Breakdown Cycle, which you were in before you started your reset.

The Optimized Nutrition Plan generates exceptional energy to meet your daily demands, enhances your fitness levels, and creates that ideal body you've been dreaming about. Are you ready to go the next level?

If so, then it's important to understand that long-term compliance is critical for success in this phase. The program is sustainable for true long-term progress, and if you follow it, you will reap the rewards for your efforts year after year, constantly reaching new heights.

The Optimized Nutrition Plan should be your year-round nutrition plan except for 3 weeks each year when I recommend you do the 21-Day Reset. If you fall off the program after spending a long weekend in Vegas or taking a vacation, I've created a 7-day reboot to get you back on track.

How High-Performance Optimized Nutrition Works

Reintroduction of Eliminated Foods

During the Reset, I know you may have started to miss or crave foods that were not on the approved-foods list. Hey, I get it. Food tastes good, especially the foods you're fond of. That's why now I'm giving you the option of reintroducing some of those foods to see if they can fit back into your diet without causing food-induced inflammation, intolerance, and discomfort or leading you back into the Metabolic Breakdown Cycle. You don't really want to go back to feeling like that, do you?

Look, if you are feeling great by sticking with the current approved-foods list, then there is no need to reintroduce anything. "If it ain't broke, don't fix it!"

However, if you find yourself craving foods that are not on the approved-foods list, go ahead and make a list of the foods you miss most. Reintroduce the foods *one by one,* following this simple re-introduction protocol:

- Choose *one* food to reintroduce.

- Consume significant servings of the reintroduced food on day 1 (for example, if you want to reintroduce dairy, have yogurt and a glass of milk at breakfast and large glasses of milk at lunch and dinner). Then abstain from the food for at least 2 days following to allow time for delayed-response symptoms to appear. Without this time period, you might miss sensitivity signs.

- During days 2 and 3, mark any of the following symptoms that occur:

  ☐ *Insomnia*   ☐ *Itching in the roof*
  ☐ *Bloating*   *of your mouth*
  ☐ *Constipation*   ☐ *Gas or belching*
  ☐ *Acid reflux*   ☐ *Diarrhea*
  ☐ *Allergies*   ☐ *Joint pain*
  ☐ *Wired at night*   ☐ *Sneezing*
  ☐ *Foggy thinking*   ☐ *Fatigue*
  ☐ *Loss of libido*   ☐ *Wheezing*
  ☐ *Ringing in ears*   ☐ *Runny nose*
  ☐ *Headaches*   ☐ *Intense cravings*
  ☐ *Puffy, watery, or itchy eyes*

- If you experience any of these symptoms, you need to eliminate that food from your diet again.

- If on days 2 and 3 you experienced no symptoms, you can occasionally include the trial food back into your diet.

You must follow this protocol on all the nonapproved foods you miss to make sure you do not reintroduce a food that causes inflammation back into your diet.

Optimized Eating

Next, we want to make sure you are eating foods that enhance and maintain *optimized metabolic resiliency, high energy, charged sex drive,* and *deep, regenerative sleep.*

Eat protein and vegetables at every meal. Protein and vegetables are the core of the Optimized Nutrition Plan. They must be consumed at every meal. They provide the building blocks for all the chemical reactions, hormones, neurotransmitters, and tissues within the body that make up the metabolism; without them health is compromised and true metabolic resiliency cannot be developed.

Eat ample amounts of healthy fats. Healthy fats enhance brain function and provide support for hormone development. Eating fat earlier in the day stabilizes blood sugar, controls food cravings, and improves your ability to lose body fat. Fat is also a great way to wake the brain up and support drive and focus, helping you to become a production machine. Fat helps us look good, generates our mojo, and keeps us focused to make smart decisions, and it's essential to your long-term success.

Consume complex carbohydrates. Skip the carbs, and your metabolism will stall out quickly and your results will quickly diminish. Furthermore, *the more you exercise, the more carbohydrates you need.*

When you exercise, you deplete muscle glycogen. Glycogen comes from carbohydrates. When glycogen starts running low and isn't being replaced from carbohydrate consumption, you will experience fatigue, lack of motivation, and a noticeable decrease in performance. Not good!

I am not proposing that you become a carboholic, as that can lead to a whole cascade of different health problems, but you do need to recognize that carbohydrates are a serious piece of the Optimized Nutrition protocol and must be included in your diet if you want to maintain and optimize your progress.

Research shows that if you follow a calorie-restricted or low-carbohydrate diet for too long, your metabolism begins to slow down. The human body is a highly adaptive organism and eventually responds to these restrictions by downregulating a hormone called leptin. Reduced leptin levels increase hunger and cravings while slowing the metabolic rate and reducing energy expenditure—not a good combo. In addition, leptin is a master control hormone, meaning its levels have an effect on other hormones such as testosterone, growth hormone, and thyroid hormones. Lower levels of these hormones cause your metabolism to be sluggish and leave you looking and feeling lousy and hungry.

So what's the answer?

Here it comes.

It's called *carbohydrate cycling.*

Carbohydrate cycling is a method of eating carbohydrates that enhances performance and does not increase the risk of type 2 diabetes, heart disease, or other health problems associated with high levels of carb intake. Carbohydrate cycling means consuming a modest amount of carbs daily for 6 days a week and then on the 7th day including a Metabolic Boost high-carb cheat meal (200–300 grams; for ready-made foods you can check the label for number of grams of carbs). Think of it as a cheat meal that improves how you look, recover, and perform.

For example, for most of the week I consume 80–120 grams of carbs daily, about 2 cups of complex carbs like rice or sweet potatoes. Then on the 7th day a typical Metabolic Boost meal for me consists of 3 gluten-free pancakes with 4–5 tablespoons of blueberry syrup, followed by 3–5 ounces of gluten- and dairy-free frozen yogurt. Notice that I stay gluten-free and dairy-free for my Metabolic Boost meal. When I reintroduced gluten and dairy, they caused me lots of problems, so I leave them out. If you have reintroduced either of those and not had a negative response, you can include gluten- and dairy-based foods in this meal.

Carb cycling has been around for years in the body-transformation and body-building realms. It's one of the reasons body builders can get their body-fat levels down so low. They learned early on that low-carb or no-carb diets will only reduce body fat for a very short time and lead to lethargy. But by carb cycling with a Metabolic Boost high-carb meal, they not only burn fat, but feel great.

Having a larger than normal meal with lots of carbohydrates causes leptin and other hormones to spike, kick-starting your metabolism back into high gear, so you can continue to feel great, look great, and perform great. These simple Metabolic Boost meals once a week are the key to keeping your metabolism supercharged and resilient. They also give you an opportunity to eat and enjoy the foods you love, but aren't able to include during the rest of the week.

The outcome of eating to optimize your metabolism is a resilient, energetic, lean, sexy, incredibly motivated *you*!

Athletes and lean people (can-see-your-abs lean) who exercise at a high intensity more than 4 days a week will need to consume even more carbohydrates during the Metabolic Boost meal. Aim for 400–600 grams of carbs during the Metabolic Boost meal. Your carbohydrate intake during the week can also increase. I have found 200 grams a day to be more ideal. If your body fat is below 8 percent, you will want to have the Metabolic Boost meal twice a week.

The Twelve Lifestyle Modifications for the Stark Naked High-Performance Optimized Nutrition Plan

1. Coffee is back. Yeah!!! Yes, you read that right! You can have coffee again. I personally love coffee. I like to pretend I am a coffee connoisseur and roast my own beans. I love every part of coffee—the smell, the taste, the experience—so removing coffee is the toughest part of the 21-Day Reset for me. So of course I have figured out how to work it back into our lives. If you are enjoying the green tea you've been drinking, you do not have to switch back to coffee, but if you miss coffee as much as I do during the Reset, please feel free to reintroduce it and pray it doesn't make you feel bad. However, you need to make sure you control your intake. Limit coffee to 1 12-ounce cup a day, and I highly recommend you get the best-quality coffee you can find. Coffee crops are heavily sprayed with pesticides, so go organic whenever possible.

2. It's okay to enjoy up to 4 glasses of wine throughout the week.

Wow! Brad is recommending coffee and alcohol? I love this guy, but what's the catch?

Hey, I enjoy a glass of wine with my wife. I love the alone time to reconnect with her, and of course what usually follows wine consumption. Thanks to my increased mojo, so does she! I would rather have you enjoy a glass of wine and decompress from all the stimulation of the world than stare at your TV or computer. We need more connection with other human beings as much as we need more sleep. Enjoying a glass of wine together is one way to create that connection. So if you drink, go ahead and enjoy wine with friends or loved ones a couple of times a week.

I prefer red wine as the optimal choice, because the resveratrol found in red wine enhances insulin sensitivity, making it less likely you will get fat from the increased carbohydrate intake. Just keep it to a max of 2 glasses in a day. The key here is control. Less is always more.

3. Continue to keep refined sugar to a minimum.

It's okay to enjoy a little refined sugar during your Metabolic Boost meal, but try to keep it to a minimum the rest of the week. Sugar is essentially empty calories that do nothing good for the body and have actually been shown to lead to nutrient deficiencies. Sugar in the form of fructose is needed by the liver in small amounts to replenish liver glycogen but too much consumption of it just adds extra unneeded work for your already stressed and overloaded liver. You can get enough natural fructose from a couple of servings of fruit daily.

Sugar consumption in the form of glucose causes elevations in insulin and can potentially lead to type 2 diabetes, making it almost impossible to lose weight. And if that's not enough to deter you, sugar has also been linked to cancer. There is nothing beneficial to consuming sugar outside of a little natural fructose from fruit to refill liver glycogen.

4. Avoid complex carbohydrates for breakfast. In the morning, after a night of sleeping and fasting, our insulin levels (the hormone that tells the body to store energy) are low and our muscles are full of glycogen. If you want to prevent your body from storing fat, this is not the time to eat carbs. Eating carbs at breakfast will cause an insulin spike telling your body to stop burning fat and start storing it instead. We do not want to start our day storing fat. Instead, have some fat at breakfast and your body will consume that as fuel.

According to research by Molly S. Bray, of the University of Alabama at Birmingham, mice fed a high-fat meal at the beginning of the day were able to burn fat more efficiently throughout the day, suggesting that what you eat for breakfast may dictate which energy source your body will use for the rest of the day. They were also better able to breakdown and utilize the components of a mixed diet, including carbohydrates, fats, and protein throughout the day. It is critical that you avoid complex carbohydrates for your breakfast for optimal health, performance, and fat loss.

5. Hydrate. Continue to drink half your body weight in ounces of water every day. Your trips to the bathroom should have slowed to a manageable number. If you are still taking more trips than you would like, you should really try adding ConcenTrace Trace Mineral Drops to your water.

6. Sleep 7 to 9 hours a night every night. Remember, the more complicated the brain, the more sleep you need. That is why you are going to continue to sleep for 7 to 9 hours every night. I want you in bed by no later than 11:00 P.M. if you can. Sleep recharges your battery, and it's when your body goes into healing mode! At this point sleep is critical for your long-term success and resiliency. *Do not cheat sleep!*

7. Exercise. Phase 2 is built to support a high volume of exercise, so you finally have the green light to hit it hard again. Your body is primed and ready for it, but please remember to include at least two recovery workouts a week in your program. Also unless you're a professional athlete or training for a big event like a marathon, keep your high-intensity workouts to a maximum of 4 times a week. Research has shown that training hard for a maximum of 45 minutes is ideal. If your workout takes longer than that, you're spending too much time socializing, not training.

8. Commit to daily acts of relaxation. Continue to find time to take small relaxation breaks during your day. Again, anything you find relaxing works, and it can continue to be for as little as 10 minutes. Examples are meditation, focused deep breathing, reading a book, or a 10-minute nap in the afternoon. If you haven't tried the meditation apps I discussed in Phase 1 (also see the Resource Guide), now may be a great time to experiment. Both are voice guided and do a phenomenal job of calming you down with zero effort on your part. Just sit back and let the voice lead you.

9. You're allowed to reintroduce foods. Just follow the reintroduction process laid out earlier in this chapter and pay attention to your body's response. You'll also note that there are more foods on the Phase 2 approved-foods list for you to enjoy. These foods do not require you to go through the reintroduction process.

10. Maximize protein and vegetable intake. This rule stays in effect. This is not a deprivation diet, so don't starve yourself. The protein and vegetable serving sizes are the minimums you are allowed to eat. *You can eat as much protein and as many vegetables as you want* *for lunch and dinner.* Remember, these foods possess the ultimate rebuilding blocks for your metabolism, so don't be shy.

11. Follow carbohydrate and fat servings exactly. Continue to follow these guidelines exactly as laid out. They will help you drop body fat and obtain that great-looking body you're searching for without wiping out your metabolism.

12. Stick to three meals a day, but add snacks if needed. I have added a couple of snacks to Phase 2. They are completely optional, and if you are having great success with only three meals a day, then there is no need to make any changes. However, if as your exercise volume increases your hunger increases, you may want to add a couple of small snacks to keep hunger under control, so you don't become irritable and no fun to be around.

Are you ready to take your metabolism and life to the next level?

Let's do this!

Approved Foods

PHASE 2 APPROVED FOODS
Note: If you have successfully reintroduced foods that were disallowed during Phase 1, for example, gluten, dairy, shellfish, or beans, you may add them back to the list.
Proteins
Eggs
Poultry (chicken, turkey, duck, ostrich, Cornish game hen)
Pork
Free-range beef
All fish
Wild game meats (buffalo, bison, boar, venison, antelope, duck)
Fats
Coconut oil
Olive oil

Macadamia nut oil
Walnut oil
Avocado oil
Seeds (sesame, flax, chia, hemp, pumpkin, and sunflower seeds)
Heavy whipping cream
Organic butter and ghee
Avocado
Unsweetened canned coconut milk
Unsweetened almond milk
All nuts except peanuts
Carbohydrates for Regular Meals
Rice (all types)
Potatoes (all types)
Sweet Potatoes
Yams
Quinoa
Gluten-Free Oats
Additional Carbohydrates for the Metabolic Boost Cheat Meal
Gluten-free pasta
Gluten-free pancakes and waffles
Gluten-free desserts and treats
Gluten- and dairy-free ice cream or frozen yogurt
Bananas
Grapes
Vegetables
All vegetables except carrots, beets, peas, and corn
Fruits
All fruits except bananas and grapes
Herbs and Spices
All herbs and spices
Beverages
Water
Green tea
Herbal teas
Coffee (1 12-ounce cup max daily)

Meals and Serving Sizes

PHASE 2 DAILY OUTLINE	
Hydration	
Number of ounces of water that equals half your body weight throughout the day	
Upon Waking	
6 ounces warm water with juice from ½ lemon (optional)	
Breakfast (within 1 hour of waking)	
Men	2 servings protein, 2 servings fat, 1 serving coffee*
Women	1 serving protein, 1 serving fat, 1 serving coffee*
Mid-Morning Snack	
1 serving fruit, 1 serving nuts or other fat, or 1 detox smoothie (optional)	
Lunch	
Men	2 servings protein, 2 servings vegetables, 2 servings fat*
Women	1 serving protein, 2 servings vegetables, 1 serving fat*
Mid-Afternoon Snack	
1 serving fruit or 1 serving nuts or other fat (optional)	
Dinner	
Men	2 servings protein, 2 servings vegetables, 2 servings fat, 3 servings carbs*
Women	1 serving protein, 2 servings vegetables, 1 serving fat, 2 servings carbs*
Before-Bed Snack	
1 serving tryptophan-enhancing food: ½ cup full-fat cottage cheese, a handful of cashews, a handful of pecans, 1 scoop whey protein powder, dark chocolate	
Weekly Carbohydrate Cycling Instructions	
One night a week consume a high-carbohydrate cheat meal that includes 200–300 grams of carbohydrates. Red wine is allowed with this meal (2 glasses max).	
*Note: Just as in Phase 1, protein and vegetable servings are minimums with no maximums.	

SERVING SIZES	
Protein	1 serving = 3 ounces uncooked meat (about the size of a deck of cards), 2 whole eggs
Vegetables	1 serving = 1 cup raw
Fat	1 serving = 1 tablespoon oil, butter, heavy whipping cream, ½ avocado, ¼ cup seeds, ¼ cup nuts
Carbohydrates	1 serving = 1 cup *cooked*
Fruit	1 serving = ½ cup

Phase 2: 7-Day Sample Meal Plan

Below is a sample 7-day meal plan for Phase 2. As in the Reset, as long as you stick with the approved foods and nutritional requirements, meals can be as basic or as gourmet as you like. Use the recipes from Chapter 12 as a starting point. Pay attention to the servings of fats, carbs, and fruits in each recipe and adjust as needed to fit your requirements. Remember, you can eat as much protein and vegetables as you want.

	Breakfast	Morning Snack	Lunch	Afternoon Snack	Dinner	Bedtime
PHASE 2 SAMPLE MEAL PLAN						
Day 1	Eggs Cooked in Coconut Oil Avocado	Apple Cashews	Mini Meatloaf Raw Kale and Brussels Sprout Salad	Apple Cashews Green Tea	Halibut Tacos with Jicama Shells and Cilantro Slaw	Cottage Cheese
Day 2	Create Your Own Protein Shake	Raspberries Almonds	Shredded Pork Lettuce Wraps	Raspberries Almonds Green Tea	Hearty Bison Stew	Cashews
Day 3	Sautéed Ground Buffalo Macadamia Nuts	Mixed Berries Heavy Cream	Kabobs with Chimichurri Sauce Roasted Vegetables	Mixed Berries Heavy Cream Green Tea	Yam, Chicken, and Kale Stir-Fry	Pecans

	Breakfast	Morning Snack	Lunch	Afternoon Snack	Dinner	Bedtime
Day 4	Eggs cooked in Coconut Oil Avocado	Plum Walnuts	Fajita Bowl with Pico de Gallo Salad with Avocado Dressing	Plums Walnuts Green Tea	Turkey Sliders with Pickled Red Onions Yam or Sweet Potato Fries	Dark Chocolate
Day 5	Sautéed Ground Beef Avocado	Pineapple Cashews	Ground Chicken Lettuce Wraps Creamed Veggie Soup	Pineapple Cashews Green Tea	Asian Meatballs Kicked-Up Quinoa Salad	Cherries
Day 6	Create Your Own Protein Shake	Apple Almonds	Bison Meatballs with San Marzano Sauce Roasted Vegetables	Apple Almonds Green Tea	Sea Bass with Garlic, Ginger, and Coconut Oil Coconut-Ginger Rice	Cottage Cheese
Day 7	Sautéed Ground Turkey Nitrate-Free Bacon	Mixed Berries Heavy Cream	Mini Meatloaf Creamed Veggie Soup	Mixed Berries Heavy Cream Green Tea	Moussaka	Cashews

You can have up to 2 protein smoothies for breakfast each week during Phase 2. Make sure to follow these steps. Follow the serving-size guidelines for the appropriate amount of each ingredient to add.

PHASE 2 SHAKES: CREATE YOUR OWN	
Choose a Protein Powder	
Serving size: 1 scoop for women, 2 scoops for men	
Whey protein	Vegan protein (rice, pea, hemp)
Choose a Green	
Serving size: approximately 2 handfuls	
Kale	Spinach
Romaine	Arugula
Cabbage	Lettuce
Chard	Collard greens
Choose a Fruit	
Serving size: 1 cup max	
Pineapple	Mango

Papaya	Green apple
Lemon	Lime
Berries (any type except blueberries)	
Choose a Healthy Fat	
Serving size: Amounts listed are for women. Double for men.	
½ avocado	Coconut oil, 1 tablespoon
Organic butter, 1 tablespoon	Heavy whipping cream, 1 tablespoon
Unsweetened canned coconut milk, ½ cup	Olive oil, 1 tablespoon
Choose a Veggie Boost for Taste (Optional)	
Serving size: as desired	
Celery	Cucumber
Bell pepper	Parsley
Mint	Ginger root (use a small amount)
Dandelion root (use a small amount)	Jalapeños (use a small amount)
Choose a Superfood (Optional)	
Serving size: 1 teaspoon (or follow package directions)	
Cinnamon: Enhances insulin sensitivity and supports healthy blood sugar	
Maca: A natural adaptogen helping the body to adapt to stress; also a natural hormone balancer; increases energy and promotes a healthy sex drive	
Cacao: One of the foods richest in magnesium (supports mood, muscles, sleep, and bowel movements) and in antioxidants; the original form of chocolate, no added sugars or milk	
Probiotics: Enhance gut health	
Blend	
Blend ingredients until smooth, adding water and/or ice to reach the desired consistency.	

The 7-Day Reboot

I totally understand how life gets in the way at times or we make choices that negatively affect our metabolism. I recently volunteered to help Joseph, our eleven-year-old son, with his sixth-grade science-fair project. I was so proud that he wanted to do his project on how food affects the human body. He recruited a trainer I work with at

Stark to eat home-cooked meals for 5 days, and I agreed to be the fast-food test subject eating nothing but fast food and drinking soda for 5 days.

At first glance, it sounded like a fun cheat week, but after the second day of Joseph's experiment, my body started to rebel. I couldn't sleep, my brain felt as if it had stopped working, I was severely constipated, and every time I tried to workout I ended up throwing up. I threw in the towel after 4 days, because the food I was eating was wreaking havoc on my work and family life, not to mention my body.

I was far from a fun person to be around when I was feeling that gross. A 7-Day Reboot was the answer. I followed the Phase 1 Reset for 7 days, got back on track, and then went back to the Phase 2 Optimized Nutrition Plan. I can proudly say that after the dust settled, Joseph's experiment was definitely worth the sacrifice. He ended up being the only kid in his class to get an A+ on his science project—and it confirmed for me just how important it is to eat to support a healthy metabolism.

If you drink a little too much wine on a vacation to Napa Valley or enjoy a few too many desserts over the holidays, don't stress! Reboot when you get home. Crazy bachelor or bachelorette party in Vegas? No sweat! Enjoy the party, but come home and commit to doing the Reboot.

Life should be lived, not just endured. Have fun when you get the opportunity, and then reboot to bring your metabolism back online.

Don't beat yourself up for enjoying the finer things in life. I give you permission to fully enjoy your vacations and special occasions with friends and family. Reboot and pick right back up where you left off. If you've done the 21-Day Reset and been following the Optimized Nutrition Plan, your healthy metabolism has the resiliency to survive some fun.

The Stark Naked 21-Day Metabolic Reset Resource Guide

Safe Hygiene Products

In Chapters 3 and 5 we explored how the products that come into contact with our skin on a daily basis might be wreaking havoc on our livers and disrupting our hormones. To help you find some alternatives to the products you are currently using, I've put together a list of my favorite and safest products, including personal-care products, sunscreens, household solvents, and cleaners. If you don't find what you're looking for here, you can expand your own search at www .ewg.org.

Adult Body Wash

Dr. Bronner's 18 in 1 Hemp Pure Castile Liquid Soap
  (www.drbronner.com)
Be Green Bath and Body Bath and Shower Gel
  (www.begreenbathandbody.com)
Lion Bear Naked Soap Head to Toe Wash (www.lionbearnaked.com)

Kid's Body Wash

Dr. Robin for Kids Body Wash and Shampoo (www.dermstore.com;
search "Dr. Robin")

Healing Scents Just for Kids, Shampoo/Bath/Shower Soap
(www.healing-scents.com)

Baby Needs

Ava Anderson (www.avaandersonnontoxic.com)

Be Green Bath and Body (www.begreenbathandbody.com)

Nurture My Body (www.nurturemybody.com)

Lotion

Be Green Day Face and Hand Cream (www.begreenbathandbody.com)

Nurture My Body Moisturizer (www.nurturemybody.com)

Adult Shampoo/Conditioner

Nurture My Body Shampoo and Conditioner
(www.nurturemybody.com)

Penny Lane Organics Shampoo with Conditioner
(www.pennylaneorganics.com)

Kid's Shampoo

Dr. Robin for Kids Body Wash and Shampoo (www.dermstore.com;
search "Dr. Robin")

Healing Scents Just for Kids, Shampoo/Bath/Shower Soap
(www.healing-scents.com)

Deodorant

Jungle Man Deodorant (www.junglemannaturals.com)

Jungle Woman Deodorant (www.junglemannaturals.com)
(Trust me on these, I searched endlessly for a safe, quality
deodorant that actually worked, and this one is amazing for
both men and women!)

Adult Sunscreen

All Terrain AquaSport SPF 30 (www.allterrainco.com)
Aubrey Organics Natural Sun Sunscreen
  (www.aubrey-organics.com)

Kid's Sunscreen

Dr. Robin for Kids Sunscreen (www.dermstore.com;
  search "Dr. Robin")
Thinkbaby Sunscreen (www.gothinkbaby.com)

Household Cleaners

Green Shield Organic (www.greenshieldorganic.com)
Sun & Earth (www.sunandearth.com)
Earth Friendly Products (www.ecos.com)

Air Fresheners

Earth Friendly Products Uni-Fresh Air Freshener (www.ecos.com)
Aussan Natural Room Odor Eliminator (www.aussannatural.com)

Bulletproof Mindset Training

In Chapters 1 and 6 we explored stress and how it can lead to adrenal burnout. Below are my favorite resources, the ones I have personally used to conquer my response to mental/emotional stress, and I know they can help you battle this aspect of stress too. This collection of books, tools, and seminars has helped me reign in my inner Hulk and control my emotional response to nondangerous stressors that can literally wipe out my energy, desire for life, and sex drive.

Books

Brené Brown, *Daring Greatly: How the Courage to Be Vulnerable Transforms the Way We Live, Love, Parent, and Lead*

Mark Divine, *The Way of the SEAL: Think Like an Elite Warrior to Lead and Succeed*

Brian Klemmer, *The Compassionate Samurai: Being Extraordinary in an Ordinary World*

Bruce McEwen, with Elizabeth Norton Lasley, *The End of Stress as We Know It*

Robert Sapolsky, *Why Zebras Don't Get Ulcers*

Hans Selye, *The Stress of Life*

James L. Wilson, *Adrenal Fatigue: The 21st Century Stress Syndrome*

Tools

HeartMath Inner Balance App or emWave2 (www.heartmath.com)
These are an incredible tools using biofeedback to help you take control of your emotional states. You will learn how to transform feelings of anger, anxiety, or frustration into feelings that are more peaceful and relaxed and discover what it feels like to shut down your inner Hulk. I spent a lot of my time early on dealing with stress by using the emWave2. I literally had to reteach my brain how to calm down; I was stuck in a constant state of high stress even when I was trying to relax.

Calm App (www.calm.com)
This app for your smartphone is a great tool to relax your body, especially when you are feeling tense from stress. You can also access the Calm program on the website if you don't have a smart-phone. Just plug a pair of headphones into your computer and calm away. The program is voice-guided and does a phenomenal job getting the mind settled and quiet with minimal effort; all you have to do is just sit back and let the voice take you there. I personally use this app two to three times a day to keep my inner Hulk from emerging. (I won't lie. Every once in a while he still shows up, but I have found a way to control him 95 percent of the time, and this is one of my secrets.)

Headspace App (www.headspace.com)

This is another app for your smartphone that is a great tool for meditation. By walking you through 10 minutes a day of meditation, Andy Puddicombe helps you create a mindful meditation practice. I prefer to do the headspace program first thing every morning. I have found that starting my day with just 10 minutes of meditation clears my mind and makes me so much more effective, especially when speaking.

Seminars

Driven for Life (www.drivenforlife.com)

Driven for Life has a special place in my heart. I have attended multiple full-immersion retreats with this group, and the impact it has had on my life has been amazing. Sometimes the way to become more resilient to stress is to get out of your comfort zone and break through whatever is holding you back from living at your ultimate level. The courses offered by this group are full-immersion, detached from the rest of the world, and they really dig deep to help you grow from the inside out. Awesome life-changing experiences!

Klemmer and Associates (www.klemmer.com)

The Klemmer and Associates workshops are incredible for helping you to strip away self-doubt and the destructive belief systems that are holding you back in life and replace them with productive, beneficial, and supportive beliefs. It's amazing how much easier life is when you remove limiting beliefs. So much of the mental/emotional stress in our lives is produced by our own self-created negative belief systems.

Acknowledgments

WANT TO START by thanking Tom Ferry for taking four hours out of his busy life two years ago to coach me into thinking bigger. Your introduction to Laura Morton has forever changed the trajectory of my life. I owe a huge thank-you to my writing partner, Laura, for believing in my message, pushing me beyond my limits, and always having my back. You have been an amazing rock of stability through this process and your ability to add sizzle to my words has been amazing to witness.

Thanks to my agent, Mel Berger at William Morris Endeavor, for taking a risk with me and seeing the possibility in my work, and to Nancy Hancock, who first saw something special in my ideas and made my dream of writing a book a reality at HarperOne.

A huge shout-out and thank-you to my incredible publishing team at HarperOne, including my publisher, Mark Tauber, my amazing editor, Julia Pastore, and the entire production, marketing, publicity, and sales staff. Thank you so much for your amazing support and patience. I wish to also thank Tina Andreadis, SVP of Publicity at Harper-Collins, for all her wonderful support and belief in my program.

I am grateful for Heidi Krupp and Darren Lisiten from Krupp Kommunications for their guidance in getting my message out to the world.

I want to thank my business partner, Todd Vande Hei, for his amazing support and for guiding our company into a position that would allow me to focus on writing this book. Thank you to the amazing staff at Stark: you are truly the heart and soul of this message and I love watching you all touch and change lives on a daily basis. Thank you to our clients, who have put their faith and trust in our programs, and thank you to all those courageous souls who willingly tested the Stark Naked 21-Day Metabolic Reset. Your experiences helped me to shape and perfect this program; I could not have completed this without your bravery.

Deep gratitude goes to all of the mentors I have had through the years who have taken the time to offer me guidance, counsel, and support on my journey.

Thank you to my amazing friends who have always been there for me throughout the years, with an extra special thank-you to three of the greatest friends a guy could ask for, Jason Von, Jeff Stover, and Chris Panaia. Thank you for being there through thick and thin—your friendships I will always cherish.

To my family: I am forever grateful for your support and belief in me. Maria and my kiddos, you have given my life incredible meaning.

Mom and Dad, thank you for always being there to pick me up, brush me off, and kick me in my fanny to keep moving forward.

Jake and Katie, life growing up with you was amazing. I so cherish the times our families get together. To my extended family, thank you for all your support, and to my wife's family here in California, thank you so much for the support during the writing of this book. Without your help with our kids, this book would never have reached completion!

Bibliography

Afaghi, Ahmad, Helen O'Connor, and Chin Moi Chow. "High-glycemic-index Carbohydrate Meals Shorten Sleep Onset." *American Journal of Clinical Nutrition* 85(2) (February 2007): 426–30. http://ajcn.nutrition.org/content/85/2/426.full.pdf.

Alter, Charlotte. "Going Off the Pill Could Affect Who You're Attracted to, Study Finds." *Time*. November 20, 2014. http://time.com/3596014/attraction-sex-birth-control/.

Amen, Daniel G. *Change Your Brain, Change Your Life: The Breakthrough Program for Conquering Anxiety, Depression, Obsessiveness, Anger, and Impulsiveness*. New York: Three Rivers, 1998.

American College of Cardiology. "Low LDL Cholesterol Is Related to Cancer Risk." *ScienceDaily*. March 26, 2012. www.sciencedaily.com/releases/2012/03/120326113713.htm.

"Androgen Deficiency in Women." *Better Health Channel*. October 22, 2014. www.betterhealth.vic.gov.au/bhcv2/bhcarticles.nsf/pages/Androgen_deficiency_in_women.

Angelilli, Jonathan. "The Massive Fitness Trend That's Not Actually Healthy at All." *Greatist*. September 29, 2014. http://greatist.com/connect/militarization-fitness.

Anwar, Yasmin. "Sleep Deprivation Linked to Junk Food Cravings." *UC Berkeley NewsCenter*. August 6, 2013. http://newscenter.berkeley.edu/2013/08/06/poor-sleep-junk-food/.

Aude, Y. Wady, et al. "The National Cholesterol Education Program Diet vs. a Diet Lower in Carbohydrates and Higher in Protein and Monounsaturated Fat." *Archives of Internal Medicine* 164(19) (October 25, 2004): 2141–46. http://archinte.jamanetwork.com/article.aspx?articleid=217514.

Bannai, Makoto, and Nobuhiro Kawai. "New Therapeutic Strategy for Amino Acid Medicine: Glycine Improves the Quality of Sleep." *Journal of Pharmacological Sciences* 118(2) (2012): 145–48. www.ncbi.nlm.nih.gov/pubmed/22293292.

Barrett-Connor, Elizabeth, et al. "The Association of Testosterone Levels with Overall Sleep Quality, Sleep Architecture, and Sleep-Disordered Breathing." *Journal of Clinical Endocrinology and Metabolism* 93(7) (July 2008): 2602–9. www.ncbi.nlm.nih.gov/pmc/articles/PMC2453053/.

Belluck, Pam. "In Study, Fatherhood Leads to Drop in Testosterone." *New York Times.* September 12, 2011. www.nytimes.com/2011/09/13/health/research/13testosterone.html ?_r=0.

Bennington, Vanessa. "How Sleep Deprivation Fries Your Hormones, Your Immune System, and Your Brain." *Breaking Muscle.* http://breakingmuscle.com/health-medicine /how-sleep-deprivation-fries-your-hormones-your-immune-system-and-your-brain.

Berardi, John. "The Get Shredded Diet." *T Nation.* July 10, 2006. http://www.t-nation.com /diet-fat-loss/the-get-shredded-diet.

"The Best Foods for Your Brain." *Prevention.* March 28, 2014. www.prevention.com/food /healthy-eating-tips/best-foods-your-brain.

"Bisphenol A (BPA)." *Breast Cancer Fund.* www.breastcancerfund.org/clear-science /radiation-chemicals-and-breast-cancer/bisphenol-a.html.

Blank, M. C., et al. "Total Body Na-depletion without Hyponatraemia Can Trigger Overtraining-like Symptoms with Sleeping Disorders and Increasing Blood Pressure: Explorative Case and Literature Study." *Medical Hypotheses* 79(6) (2012): 799–804. www.ncbi.nlm.nih.gov/pubmed/23234732.

Bledzka, Dorota, Jolanta Gromadzinska, and Wojciech Wasowicz. "Parabens: From Environmental Studies to Human Health." *Environment International* 67 (2014): 27–42. www.ncbi.nlm.nih.gov/pubmed/24657492.

"Body Burden: The Pollution in Newborns." *Environmental Working Group.* July 14, 2005. www.ewg.org/research/body-burden-pollution-newborns.

Boyles, Salynn. "Estrogen Is Involved in Stress Response." *WebMD.* December 3, 2003. www.webmd.com/depression/news/20031203/estrogen-is-involved-in-stress-response.

Brehm, Bonnie, et al. "A Randomized Trial Comparing a Very Low Carbohydrate Diet and a Calorie-Restricted Low Fat Diet on Body Weight and Cardiovascular Risk Factors in Healthy Women." *Journal of Clinical Endocrinology and Metabolism* 88(4) (2013): 1617–23. http://press.endocrine.org/doi/citedby/10.1210/jc.2002-021480.

Breus, Michael. "Early Bird or Night Owl? It's in Your Genes." December 14, 2012. www .psychologytoday.com/blog/sleep-newzzz/201212/early-bird-or-night-owl-it-s-in-your -genes.

———. "Mind-body Therapies to Ease Insomnia." Insomnia Blog. *Sleep Doctor.* November 6, 2014. www.theinsomniablog.com/the_insomnia_blog/2014/11/mind-body-therapies -to-ease-insomnia.html.

———. "Sports' Secret Weapon: Sleep." Insomnia Blog. *Sleep Doctor.* November 19, 2012. www.theinsomniablog.com/the_insomnia_blog/2012/11/sports-secret-weapon-sleep .html.

Burke, Leo. "Quotations About Sleep." www.quotegarden.com/sleep.html.

"Can't Sleep? Neither Can 60 Million Other Americans." *NPR.* May 20, 2008. www.npr.org /templates/story/story.php?storyId=90638364.

Chapman, Karina (AlohaKarina). "The Importance of Play . . . for Adults." *The Positive Page.* March 7, 2012. http://thepositivepage.com/2012/03/07/the-importance-of-play -for-adults/.

Chaput, J. P., and A. Tremblay. "Sleeping Habits Predict the Magnitude of Fat Loss in Adults

Exposed to Moderate Caloric Restriction." *Obesity Facts* 5(4) (2012): 561–66. www.ncbi .nlm.nih.gov/pubmed/22854682.

Clark, Kevin. "Sleeping Your Way to the Top." *Wall Street Journal.* November 14, 2012. www.wsj.com/articles/SB10001424127887324556304578117112742606502.

Conger, Cristen. "5 Ways Birth Control Can Trip Up Your Love Life." *HowStuffWorks.* February 6, 2012. http://health.howstuffworks.com/sexual-health/contraception/5-ways -birth-control-affects-love-life.htm#page=0.

Craig, B. W., R. Brown, and J. Everhart. "Effects of Progressive Resistance Training on Growth Hormone and Testosterone Levels in Young and Elderly Subjects." *Mechanisms of Ageing and Development* 49(2) (1989): 159–69. www.ncbi.nlm.nih.gov /pubmed/2796409.

Croson, Eastan. "Increasing Sleep Deprivation Rates Harm Students' Health." *SMU Daily Campus.* May 4, 2014. www.smudailycampus.com/lifestyle/health/increasing-sleep -deprivation-rates-harm-students-health.

Dean, Carolyn. "Just Say No to Birth Control Pills." *Mercola.com.* October 27, 2004. http:// articles.mercola.com/sites/articles/archive/2004/10/27/birth-control-part-two.aspx.

Dement, William C., and Charles Vaughan. *The Promise of Sleep: A Pioneer in Sleep Medicine Explores the Vital Connection Between Health, Happiness, and a Good Night's Sleep.* New York: Delacorte, 1999.

Dingfelder, Sadie. "4 of Play's Lesser-Known Benefits." *Huffington Post.* www.huffington post.com/sadie-dingfelder/play-health-benefits_b_2010275.html.

Divine, Mark. *The Way of the SEAL: Think Like an Elite Warrior to Lead and Succeed.* White Plains, NY: Reader's Digest Association, 2013.

Durmer, Jeffrey, and David Dinges. "Neurocognitive Consequences of Sleep Deprivation." *Seminars in Neurology* 25(1) (March 2005): 117–29. http://faculty.vet.upenn.edu/uep /user_documents/dfd3.pdf.

Elias, Nina. "Drink This, Sleep 90 More Minutes a Night." *Prevention.* www.prevention .com/health/sleep-energy/tart-cherry-juice-increases-sleep-time.

Epel, E. S., et al. "Stress and Body Shape: Stress-induced Cortisol Secretion Is Consistently Greater Among Women with Central Fat." *Psychosomatic Medicine* 62(5) (September–October 2000): 623–32. www.ncbi.nlm.nih.gov/pubmed/11020091.

"Erectile Dysfunction Drugs Market Is Expected to Reach USD 3.4 Billion Globally in 2019: Transparency Market Research." *PR Newswire.* October 21, 2013. www.prnewswire .com/news-releases/erectile-dysfunction-drugs-market-is-expected-to-reach-usd-34 -billion-globally-in-2019-transparency-market-research-228593931.html.

Ericsson, K. A., R. Th. Krampe, and C. Tesch-Romer. "The Role of Deliberate Practice in the Acquisition of Expert Performance." *Psychological Review* 100(3) (1993): 363–406.

Fleet, Anna. "10 Signs of Low Testosterone in Women." *ActiveBeat.* December 30, 2013. http://m.activebeat.com/your-health/women/10-signs-of-low-testosterone-in-women/.

FPS Team. "High Cholesterol and Metabolism." *Functional Performance Systems.* December 28, 2012. www.functionalps.com/blog/2010/12/28/high-cholesterol-and-metabolism/.

Frangoul, Anmar. "The World's 10 Leading Causes of Death." *CNBC.* February 6, 2014. www.cnbc.com/id/101388499/page/11.

Gittleman, Ann Louise. *The Fat Flush Plan*. New York: McGraw-Hill, 2002.

Gold, Lois, Bruce Ames, and Thomas Slone. "Misconceptions About the Causes of Cancer." In Dennis J. Paustenbach, ed., *Human and Environmental Risk Assessment: Theory and Practice*. New York: Wiley, 2002. Pp. 1415–60.

Gregoire, Carolyn. "Taking a Walk in Nature Could Be the Best Thing You Do for Your Mood All Day." *Huffington Post*. September 23, 2014. www.huffingtonpost .com/2014/09/23/walk-nature-depression_n_5870134.html.

———. "10 Ways Stress Affects Women's Health." *Huffington Post*. February 6, 2013. www .huffingtonpost.com/2013/01/30/health-effects-of-stress-women_n_2585625.html.

Grossman, Richard. "Healing Points." 1994. www.acudoc.com/exercise.html.

Gunnars, Kris. "Debunking the Calorie Myth—Why 'Calories In, Calories Out' Is Wrong." *Authority Nutrition*. http://authoritynutrition.com/debunking-the-calorie-myth/.

Halyburton, Angela, et al. "Low- and High-carbohydrate Weight-loss Diets Have Similar Effects on Mood but Not Cognitive Performance." *American Journal of Clinical Nutrition* 86(3) (September 2007): 580–87. http://ajcn.nutrition.org/content/86/3/580.long.

Hellmich, Nanci. "Sleep Loss May Equal Weight Gain." *USA Today*. December 6, 2004. http://usatoday30.usatoday.com/news/health/2004-12-06-sleep-weight-gain_x.htm.

"How Do Birth Control Pills Work?" *Go Ask Alice*. April 18, 2014. http://goaskalice .columbia.edu/how-do-birth-control-pills-work.

Hsu, Christine. "Nearly a Third of Americans Are Sleep Deprived." *Medical Daily*. April 27, 2012. www.medicaldaily.com/nearly-third-americans-are-sleep-deprived-240273.

"The Importance of Play for Adults." *First Things First*. http://firstthings.org/the-importance -of-play-for-adults.

"Insufficient Sleep Is a Public Health Epidemic." *Centers for Disease Control and Prevention*. January 13, 2014. www.cdc.gov/features/dssleep/.

Jones, Rachel. "Beyond Birth Control: The Overlooked Benefits of Oral Contraceptive Pills." *Guttmacher Institute*. www.guttmacher.org/pubs/Beyond-Birth-Control.pdf.

Kadey, Matthew. "The 11 Best Foods for Your Brain." *Shape Magazine*. www.shape.com /healthy-eating/diet-tips/11-best-foods-your-brain.

Kay, Vanessa, Michael Bloom, and Warren Foster. "Reproductive and Developmental Effects of Phthalate Diesters in Males." *Critical Reviews in Toxicology* 44(6) (2014): 467–98. www.ncbi.nlm.nih.gov/pubmed/24903855.

Kharrazian, Datis. *Why Isn't My Brain Working? A Revolutionary Understanding of Brain Decline and Effective Strategies to Recover Your Brain's Health*. Carlsbad, CA: Elephant Press, 2013.

Khoo, Joan, et al. "Comparing Effects of Low- and High-Volume Moderate-Intensity Exercise on Sexual Function and Testosterone in Obese Men." *Journal of Sexual Medicine* 10(7) (2013): 1823–32. www.ncbi.nlm.nih.gov/pubmed/23635309.

Kirby, Elizabeth, et al. "Stress Increases Putative Gonadotropin Inhibitory Hormone and Decreases Luteinizing Hormone in Male Rats." *Proceedings of the National Academy of Sciences* 106(27) (2009): 11324–29. www.pnas.org/content/106/27/11324.full.

Kirchhof, Mark, and Gillian De Gannes. "The Health Controversies of Parabens." *Skin Therapy Letter* 18(2) (2013): 5–7. www.ncbi.nlm.nih.gov/pubmed/23508773.

Klingmuller, D., and A. Allera. "Endocrine Disruptors: Hormone-active Chemicals from the Environment: A Risk to Humans?" *Deutsche Medizinische Wochenschrift* 136(18) (2011): 967–72. www.ncbi.nlm.nih.gov/pubmed/21526461.

Knutson, Kristen, et al. "The Metabolic Consequences of Sleep Deprivation." *Sleep Medicine Reviews* 11(3) (2007): 163–78. www.ncbi.nlm.nih.gov/pmc/articles/PMC1991337/.

Koebler, Jason. "The New Moneyball? It's Major League Sleep." *US News.* June 15, 2012. www.usnews.com/news/articles/2012/06/15/the-new-moneyball-its-major-league-sleep.

Konduracka, Ewa, Krzysztof Krzemieniecki, and Grzegorz Gajos. "Relationship Between Everyday Use Cosmetics and Female Breast Cancer." *Polskie Archiwum Medycyny Wewnetrznej* 124(5) (2012): 264–69. www.ncbi.nlm.nih.gov/pubmed/24694726.

Kuoppala, Ali. "Sleep and Testosterone: Each Hour Means 15 percent More T." *Anabolic Men.* December 14, 2014. http://anabolicmen.com/sleep-testosterone/.

"Lack of Sleep Tied to Teen Sports Injuries." *American Academy of Pediatrics.* October 21, 2012. www.aap.org/en-us/about-the-aap/aap-press-room/pages/Lack-of-Sleep-Tied-to-Teen-Sports-Injuries.aspx.

Lam, Michael. "Estrogen Dominance—Part 2." *DrLam.com.* www.drlam.com/blog/estrogen-dominance-part-2/1781/.

Lange, Claudia, Bertram Kuch, and Jorg Metzger. "Estrogenic Activity of Constituents of Underarm Deodorants Determined by E-Screen Assay." *Chemosphere* 108 (2014): 101–6. www.ncbi.nlm.nih.gov/pubmed/24875918.

Larsen, Amber. "The Role of Testosterone for the Female Athlete." *Breaking Muscle.* http://breakingmuscle.com/womens-fitness/the-role-of-testosterone-for-the-female-athlete.

LaValle, James B., with Stacy Lundin Yale. *Cracking the Metabolic Code: 9 Keys to Optimal Health.* North Bergen, NJ: Basic Health Publications, 2004.

Laverne, Lauren. "Why Play Is Important to Us All." *The Guardian.* www.theguardian.com/lifeandstyle/2014/oct/05/why-play-is-important-to-us-all-lauren-laverne.

Leosdottir, M., et al. "Dietary Fat Intake and Early Mortality Patterns—Data from the Malmö Diet and Cancer Study." *Journal of Internal Medicine* 258(2) (2005): 153–65. www.ncbi.nlm.nih.gov/pubmed/16018792.

Leproult, Rachel, et al. "Sleep Loss Results in an Elevation of Cortisol Levels the Next Evening." *Sleep* 20(10) (October 1997): 865–70. www.journalsleep.org/ViewAbstract.aspx?pid=24246

Lerchbaum, Elisabeth, et al. "Combination of Low Free Testosterone and Low Vitamin D Predicts Mortality in Older Men Referred for Coronary Angiography." *Clinical Endocrinology* 77(3) (2012): 475–83.

Lorgeril, Michel, et al. "Mediterranean Diet, Traditional Risk Factors, and the Rate of Cardiovascular Complications After Myocardial Infarction: Final Report of the Lyon Diet Heart Study." *Circulation* 99(6) (1999): 779–85. www.ncbi.nlm.nih.gov/pubmed/9989963.

"Luteinising Hormone." *You & Your Hormones.* January 7, 2015. www.yourhormones.info/hormones/luteinising_hormone.aspx.

MacLean, Christopher, et al. "Effect of the Transcendental Meditation Program on Adaptive Mechanisms: Changes in Hormone Levels and Responses to Stress After Four

Months of Practice." *Psychoneuroendocrinology* 22(4) (May 1997): 277–95. www.ncbi
.nlm.nih.gov/pubmed/9226731.

Maglione-Garves, Christine, Len Kravitz, and Suzanne Schneider. "Cortisol Connection: Tips
on Managing Stress and Weight." *Stress Cortisol Connection*. www.unm.edu/~lkravitz
/Article folder/stresscortisol.html.

Marcantel, Tina. "Hormones and How They Interact." *Dr. Tina Marcantel*. February 21,
2014. www.drmarcantel.com/hormones-and-how-they-interact/.

McEvoy, Michael. "Cholesterol: Your Body Is Incapable of Making Hormones Without It."
Metabolic Healing. April 11, 2011. http://metabolichealing.com/cholesterol-your-body
-is-incapable-of-making-hormones-without-it/.

McTiernan, Anne, et al. "Effect of Exercise on Serum Estrogens in Postmenopausal Women:
A 12-Month Randomized Clinical Trial." *Cancer Research* 64 (2004): 2923–28. http://
cancerres.aacrjournals.org/content/64/8/2923.full.pdf.

Mercola, Joseph. "9 Healthy Foods to Boost Your Brain Health." *Mercola.com*. October
31, 2013. http://articles.mercola.com/sites/articles/archive/2013/10/31/9-foods-brain
-health.aspx.

———. "Research Again Confirms Links Between Poor Sleep, Weight Gain, and Cancer."
Mercola.com. July 11, 2013. http://articles.mercola.com/sites/articles/archive/2013/07/11
/poor-sleep.aspx.

Michalsen, A., et al. "Effects of Short-Term Modified Fasting on Sleep Patterns and Daytime Vigilance in Non-Obese Subjects: Results of a Pilot Study." *Annals of Nutrition and
Metabolism* 47(5) (2003): 194–200. www.ncbi.nlm.nih.gov/pubmed/12748412.

Munsters, Marjet J. M., Wim H. M. Saris, and Anita Magdalena Hennige. "Effects of Meal
Frequency on Metabolic Profiles and Substrate Partitioning in Lean Healthy Males."
PLoS One 7(6) (2012): e38632. www.ncbi.nlm.nih.gov/pubmed/22719910.

Nagendra, Ravindra, Nirmala Maruthai, and Bindu Kutty. "Meditation and Its Regulatory
Role on Sleep." *Frontiers in Neurology* 3 (April 18, 2012): 54. www.ncbi.nlm.nih.gov
/pubmed/22529834.

Nago, Naoki, et al. "Low Cholesterol Is Associated with Mortality from Stroke, Heart Disease, and Cancer: The Jichi Medical School Cohort Study." *Japan Epidemiological Association* 21(1) (2011): 67–74. www.ncbi.nlm.nih.gov/pubmed/21160131.

Nakamura, Daichi, et al. "Bisphenol A May Cause Testosterone Reduction by Adversely
Affecting Both Testis and Pituitary Systems Similar to Estradiol." *Toxicology Letters*
194(1) (2010): 16–25. www.ncbi.nlm.nih.gov/pubmed/20144698.

National Sleep Foundation. "Facts and Stats." *DrowsyDriving.org*. http://drowsydriving.org
/about/facts-and-stats/.

Neckelmann, Dag, Arnstein Mykletun, and Alv A. Dahl. "Chronic Insomnia as a Risk Factor
for Developing Anxiety and Depression." *Sleep* 30(6) (2007): 873–80. www.journalsleep
.org/ViewAbstract.aspx?pid=26880.

Owens, Paula. "Your Hormones and Where You Store Fat." *PaulaOwens.com*. http://
thepowerof4-paula.blogspot.com/2010/10/your-hormones-where-you-store-fat.html.

Park, Alice. "Tip for Insomniacs: Cool Your Head to Fall Asleep." *Time*. June 17, 2011. http://
healthland.time.com/2011/06/17/tip-for-insomniacs-cool-your-head-to-fall-asleep/.

Penev, P. D. "Association Between Sleep and Morning Testosterone Levels in Older Men." *Sleep* 30 (4) (April 2007): 427–32. www.ncbi.nlm.nih.gov/pubmed/17520786.

"Phthalates." *Breast Cancer Fund*. www.breastcancerfund.org/clear-science/radiation -chemicals-and-breast-cancer/phthalates.html.

"Progesterone." *You & Your Hormones*. www.yourhormones.info/hormones/progesterone .aspx.

Pulsipher, Charlie. "15 Foods to Improve Your Memory Naturally and Boost Brain Power." *Sunwarrior News RSS*. October 21, 2013. www.sunwarrior.com/news/brain-foods/.

Radcliffe, Shawn. "Birth Control Pills Affect Long-Term Relationships." *Men's Fitness*. www .mensfitness.com/women/sex-tips/birth-control-pills-affect-long-term-relationships.

Reinberg, Steven. "Low Testosterone Could Increase Death Risk." *Consumer Health-Day*. August 15, 2006. http://consumer.healthday.com/general-health-information-16 /endocrinology-news-231/low-testosterone-could-increase-death-risk–534396.html.

Reynolds, Amy, et al. "Impact of Five Nights of Sleep Restriction on Glucose Metabolism, Leptin, and Testosterone in Young Adult Men." *PLOS One* 7(7) (July 23, 2012): e41218. http://journals.plos.org/plosone/article?id=10.1371/journal.pone.0041218.

Richards, Byron. "Unclog Your Liver and Lose Abdominal Fat—Leptin Diet Weight Loss Challenge #6." *Wellness Resources*. May 7, 2012. www.wellnessresources.com/weight /articles/unclog_your_liver_lose_your_abdominal_fat_leptin_diet_weight_loss _challenge/.

Ruper, Stefani. "Low on Progesterone? Why Stress Reduction Might Be the Only Way to Hack It." *Paleo for Women*. March 19, 2013. http://paleoforwomen.com/low-on -progesterone-stress-reduction-might-be-the-only-one-way-to-hack-it/.

Sapolsky, Robert. "Sex and Reproduction." In *Why Zebras Don't Get Ulcers*. 3rd ed. New York: Holt, 1994. Pp. 120–143.

Schackne, Elliott. "Fix Your Breakfast." *Orion Lifestyle*. January 15, 2015. www.orionlifestyle .com/#!Fix-Your-Breakfast/clfr/3827CC11-72A3-41EB-9F92-59F8FBDF40F1.

Schatz, Irwin, et al. "Cholesterol and All-cause Mortality in Elderly People from the Honolulu Heart Program: A Cohort Study." *Lancet* 358(9279) (August 4, 2001): 351–55. www .ncbi.nlm.nih.gov/pubmed/11502313.

Schauss, Mark. *Achieving Victory Over a Toxic World*. Bloomington, IN: Author House, 2008.

Schwarzbein, Diana, and Nancy Deville. *The Schwarzbein Principle: The Truth About Losing Weight, Being Healthy, and Feeling Younger*. Deerfield Beach, FL: Health Communications, 1999.

Scott, S. J. "How Good Habits Can Decrease Stress on Multiple Levels." *Develop Good Habits*. December 18, 2014. www.developgoodhabits.com/decreases-stress-habits/.

Seaman, Greg. "The Healing Power of a Walk in the Woods." *Eartheasy Blog*. July 5, 2011. http://eartheasy.com/blog/2011/07/the-healing-power-of-a-walk-in-the-woods/.

Shankar, Anoop, Srinivas Teppala, and Charumathi Sabanayagam. "Urinary BPA Levels and Measures of Obesity: Results from the NHANES." *ISRN Endocrinology* 2012(965423) (2012). www.ncbi.nlm.nih.gov/pubmed/22852093.

Siri-Tarino, Patty, et al. "Saturated Fat, Carbohydrate, and Cardiovascular Disease."

American Journal of Clinical Nutrition 91(3) (2010): 502–09. http://ajcn.nutrition.org/content/91/3/502.abstract.

Sisson, Mark. "Chronotypes: Are You an Early Bird or a Night Owl?" *Mark's Daily Apple*. November 5, 2013. www.marksdailyapple.com/chronotypes-are-you-an-early-bird-or-a-night-owl/#axzz2jp0zMfUI.

———. "How to Manufacture the Best Night of Sleep in Your Life." *Mark's Daily Apple*. November 6, 2013. http://www.marksdailyapple.com/how-to-manufacture-the-best-night-of-sleep-in-your-life/#axzz3NLMVL9Ti.

———. "Testosterone: Not So Manly After All?" *Mark's Daily Apple*. June 29, 2010. www.marksdailyapple.com/testosterone-women/#axzz3NDAXfiul.

———. "Your Heart Is Telling You to Sleep." *Mark's Daily Apple*. December 27, 2008. www.marksdailyapple.com/link-between-sleep-heart-health/#axzz3NLMVL9Ti.

"Sleep and Mood." *Healthy Sleep*. Division of Sleep Medicine at Harvard Medical School. http://healthysleep.med.harvard.edu/need-sleep/whats-in-it-for-you/mood.

Smith, Pamela. "A Comprehensive Look at Hormones and the Effects of Hormone Replacement." *American Academy of Anti-Aging Medicine*. www.a4m.com/assets/pdf/bookstore/aamt_vol7_41_smith.pdf.

Sondike, Stephan, Nancy Copperman, and Marc Jacobson. "Effects of a Low-carbohydrate Diet on Weight Loss and Cardiovascular Risk Factor in Overweight Adolescents." *Journal of Pediatrics* 142(3) (2003): 253–58. www.sciencedirect.com/science/article/pii/S0022347602402065.

Sprague, Brian, et al. "Circulating Serum Xenoestrogens and Mammographic Breast Density." *Breast Cancer Research* 15(3) (2013): R45. www.ncbi.nlm.nih.gov/pubmed/23710608.

Strandberg, Timo, et al. "Long-term Mortality After 5-Year Multifactorial Primary Prevention of Cardiovascular Diseases in Middle-aged Men." *Journal of the American Medical Association* 266(9) (1991): 1225–29. http://jama.jamanetwork.com/article.aspx?articleid=391550.

"Stress Effects on the Body." *American Psychological Association*. http://www.apa.org/helpcenter/stress-body.aspx.

"Survey: Americans Know How to Get Better Sleep—but Don't Act on It." *Better Sleep Council*. http://bettersleep.org/better-sleep/the-science-of-sleep/sleep-statistics-research/better-sleep-survey.

Taubes, Gary. *Why We Get Fat and What to Do About It*. New York: Knopf, 2011.

"Ten Rules for Raising Testosterone for a Stronger, Leaner Body." *Poliquin Group*. February 28, 2014. www.poliquingroup.com/ArticlesMultimedia/Articles/Article/1129/Ten_Rules_For_Raising_Testosterone_for_a_Stronger_.aspx.

Teta, Jade. "Female Belly Fat: Stress, Menopause and Other Causes." *Metabolic Effect*. June 28, 2013. www.metaboliceffect.com/female-belly-fat/.

———. "Female Hormones: Estrogen (Oestrogen) and Weight Loss." *Metabolic Effect*. June 10, 2013. www.metaboliceffect.com/female-hormones-estrogen/.

———. "Female Hormones and Weight Loss." *Metabolic Effect*. February 23, 2012. www.metaboliceffect.com/female-effect-hormones-determine-female-fat-patterns/.

———. "Hormones and Stress: Cortisol." *Metabolic Effect*. April 2, 2013. www.metabolic effect.com/hormones-stress-cortisol/.

———. "Want to Lose Fat? Count Your Hormones, Not Your Calories (Part 2)." *Huffington Post*. August 8, 2012. www.huffingtonpost.com/dr-jade-teta/weight-loss_b_1703931 .html.

Teta, Jade, and Keoni Teta. "The Calorie Trap. Why Some Will Never Win the Weight Loss Game." *Metabolic Effect*. March 1, 2012. www.metaboliceffect.com/calorie-trap-win -weight-loss-game/.

"Tip 172: Add Tart Cherries to Your Diet for Better Sleep, Better and Faster Recovery." *Poliquin Group*. September 15, 2011. www.poliquingroup.com/Tips/tabid/130 /entryid/641/Tip-172-Add-Tart-Cherries-to-Your-Diet-for-Better-Sleep-Better-and -Faster-Recovery.aspx.

"Toxin Exposure Among Children." *Unite for Sight*. www.uniteforsight.org/environmental -health/module2.

"Triazine Herbicides (Atrazine)." *Breast Cancer Fund*. www.breastcancerfund.org/clear -science/radiation-chemicals-and-breast-cancer/pesticides.html.

"The Truth About Tart Cherry Juice and Sleep." *Valley Sleep Center*. December 6, 2012. http://valleysleepcenter.com/blog/the-truth-about-tart-cherry-juice-and-sleep/.

Turner, Natasha. *The Hormone Diet: A 3-Step Program to Help You Lose Weight, Gain Strength, and Live Younger Longer*. New York: Rodale, 2010. Pp. 204–5.

Ulmer, Hanno, et al. "Why Eve Is Not Adam: Prospective Follow-up in 149,650 Women and Men of Cholesterol and Other Risk Factors Related to Cardiovascular and All-cause Mortality." *Journal of Women's Health* 13(1) (January–February 2004): 41–53. www.ncbi .nlm.nih.gov/pubmed/15006277.

Vann, Madeline. "One in Four Men Over 30 Has Low Testosterone." *ABC News*. March 23, 2015. http://abcnews.go.com/Health/Healthday/story?id=4508669.

"Vitamins and Minerals—What Do They Do?" *Netdoctor*. www.netdoctor.co.uk/health _advice/facts/vitamins_which.htm.

Volek, Jeff, Stephen Phinney, et al. "Carbohydrate Restriction Has a More Favorable Impact on the Metabolic Syndrome Than a Low-Fat Diet." *Lipids* 44(4) (2008): 297–309. http:// link.springer.com/article/10.1007/s11745-008-3274-2.

Volek, J., M. Sharman, et al. "Comparison of Energy-restricted Very Low-carbohydrate and Low-fat Diets on Weight Loss and Body Composition in Overweight Men and Women." *Nutrition and Metabolism* 1(13) (2004). www.ncbi.nlm.nih.gov/pmc/articles /PMC538279/.

Wachob, Colleen. "14 Things I Wish All Women Knew About the Pill." *MindBodyGreen*. September 13, 2013. www.mindbodygreen.com/0-10932/14-things-i-wish-all-women -knew-about-the-pill.html.

Wada, Kai, et al. "A Tryptophan-rich Breakfast and Exposure to Light with Low Color Temperature at Night Improve Sleep and Salivary Melatonin Level in Japanese Students." *Journal of Circadian Rhythms* 11(4) (May 25, 2013).

Whitman, Jessie. "The Overnight Diet: Lose Weight While You Sleep, No Exercise Required." *Fitness Watch MD*. April 18, 2013. http://fitnesswatch-md.com/2013/04/overnight-diet -lose-weight-while-you-sleep-no-exercise-required/.

Wolf, Robb. *The Paleo Solution: The Original Human Diet.* Las Vegas, NV: Victory Belt, 2010.

Wrobel, Anna, and Ewa Gregoraszczuk. "Actions of Methyl-, Propyl- and Butylparaben on Estrogen Receptor-á and -â and the Progesterone Receptor in MCF-7 Cancer Cells and Non-cancerous MCF-10A Cells." *Toxicology Letters* 230(3) (2014): 375–81. www.ncbi .nlm.nih.gov/pubmed/25128701.

Yi, S., et al. "Short Sleep Duration in Association with CT-scanned Abdominal Fat Areas: The Hitachi Health Study." *International Journal of Obesity* 37(1) (2012): 129–34. www .ncbi.nlm.nih.gov/pubmed/22349574.

"Zeranol." *Breast Cancer Fund.* www.breastcancerfund.org/clear-science/radiation -chemicals-and-breast-cancer/zeranol.html.

Zhao, Hong-yan, et al. "The Effects of Bisphenol A (BPA) Exposure on Fat Mass and Serum Leptin Concentrations Have No Impact on Bone Mineral Densities in Non-obese Pre-menopausal Women." *Clinical Biochemistry* 45(18) (December 2012): 1602–6.

Zinczenko, David. "10 Superfoods Healthier Than Kale." *Huffington Post.* December 25, 2014. www.huffingtonpost.com/david-zinczenko/10-superfoods-healthier-t_b_6213842 .html.

Index

About the Author

Brad Davidson, cofounder and performance strategist at Stark, in Irvine, California, is a highly respected nutrition and fitness expert, a world-renowned strength coach, and an international speaker on the topic of metabolism and performance enhancement. Brad grew up in the small town of McMinnville, Oregon, and moved to California in 1998 to pursue his passion for health and fitness. He opened his first Southern California gym out of his garage in 2002, and today Stark has grown into an industry leader in helping high-achieving CEOs, professional athletes, and highly driven individuals optimize their abilities to push themselves to reach their goals. Brad is currently a highly sought-after speaker for Vistage International (an executive coaching organization serving more than seventeen thousand CEOs around the world), CrossFit boxes, and sports teams throughout the United States.

Brad has trained with some of the world's leading experts in such areas as stress resiliency, cellular physiology, performance nutrition, recovery methodology, behavioral sciences, brain optimization, and hormonal regulation, leading to his development of Stark's cutting-edge protocols. He has been featured on Dr. Daniel Amen's PBS special and in his bestselling book *The Amen Solution* as the program's fitness coach and wrote the workouts for Tana Amen's bestselling book *The Omni Diet*. He was a monthly contributor to *TapOut Magazine* and *MMA Worldwide* for two years and also hosts a weekly podcast, *Stark Naked Radio*. He has also been a featured guest on the Robb Wolf Podcast and Wodcast Podcast.

Recently Brad has teamed up with Dr. Jade Teta, author, with Keoni Teta, of *The Metabolic Effect Diet* and world-renowned doctor of naturopathy, to record bimonthly video chats discussing their philosophies and answering questions from their followers related to fitness, health, nutrition, and performance. Stark serves clients from as far away as Dubai and New Zealand as well as throughout the United States and Canada.

www.braddavidson.com

Laura Morton is the coauthor of more than forty books and twenty *New York Times* bestsellers, including work with Joan Lunden, Al Roker, Melissa Etheridge, Susan Lucci, John Maxwell, Danica Patrick, Sandra Lee, Marilu Henner, Justin Bieber, and Duane "Dog" Chapman, among many others. She lives in New York.